TREATING
MARTIAL ARTS
INJURIES

BY

DENNIS R. BURKE, M.D.

Edited by Bill Griffeth

**Graphic Design and Illustration
By Walter L. Rickell**

©1981 Ohara Publications, Incorporated
All rights reserved
Printed in the United States of America
Library of Congress Catalog Card Number: 81-81332
ISBN No. 0-89750-075-X
Fifth Printing 1984

**OHARA P PUBLICATIONS, INCORPORATED
BURBANK, CALIFORNIA**

ACKNOWLEDGEMENT

A special thanks to Jane Corser, who toiled over my longhand-written pages to type the original manuscript of this book.

The editor wishes to thank Joy Denner and Tim Hazlewood for their patience during the long photo sessions, and Glendale Surgical Supplies for their invaluable help.

DEDICATION

To L.D. for the encouragement to finish this book, and to all students of the martial arts.

AUTHOR'S PREFACE

This book was written in an attempt to give the martial arts instructor and students a basic guide to recognize and treat common injuries and medical problems that are encountered in the gym and tournament area daily. There has been a need for a basic first-aid manual oriented to the specific needs of martial arts for many years. This book is not an attempt to cover every problem, only the more common. I have tried to orient the book to help the reader decide if a problem is present and whether to treat it or to refer the problem to medically-trained personnel. My background as a medical doctor with many years of experience in sports medicine (since 1962) and 13 years as an active practitioner of tae kwon do (and judo) has made a rather unique combination to produce this manual. I take no original credit except in trying to organize the book toward a martial arts outlook. The basic medical knowledge is well-known and available in many well-written manuscripts and textbooks on athletic medicine and first-aid.

Over the past several years there has been a rash of "how-to" books. It has always been my feeling that martial arts needed more how-to knowledge in dealing with common injuries that occur in training and in competition. It is hoped this small, basic-treatment manual will be kept in a handy place in the dojo or office for reference when needed. It is further hoped that the serious instructor, student and gym owner will read this book and acquaint himself with some of the basic principles in handling athletic injuries.

At the time of this writing, there are only a few early statistical studies of the prevalence and type of injuries incurred in karate-type activities. Because of this I have had to rely heavily on my own observations and experience to judge what I feel to be the more common problems. It is hoped that future studies and books on karate injuries will bear out my impressions of over 13 years experience in martial arts.

Dennis R. Burke, M.D.
Ann Arbor, Michigan

Foreword

*by Hwa Chong, 8th Dan, University of Michigan
and 1st Vice chairman,
National AAU Tae Kwon Do Committee*

All sports have a common code of sportsmanship. A martial art man's idea can be described in terms of the Oriental gentlemen: *KunJa*—the model of virtue.

In the Orient, the ultimate goal or ideal of every KunJa is to arrive at a communion with nature. KunJa is an ideal person, a man of learning and experience. A man with the virtues of wisdom or knowledge, human heartedness and courage. These virtues are defined as follows:

Chi (Wisdom): Intelligent decision and correct recognition.

Yin (Human Heartedness): It is through yin that the individual can overcome his selfishness and partiality, shed his tiny ego and unite himself with the mind of the universe which is love and creativity itself.

Through the practice of the supreme virtue of yin, man could achieve the full understanding of matters of conduct, human relations and political problems.

Yin is humanitarian love and benevolence. The man who has a compassionate heart does not worry. He who gives love always has peace of mind.

Yong (Courage): Decisive practicality; the fearlessness in action when action must be taken.

Do (The Way): The correct course which people should follow and also the principles of action, spirit and absolute goodness. Both of these are also yin. Through this do practice, we may gain virtue. In other words, the practice of do produces action which becomes virtue, yin.

The martial arts instructor should be a man of learning, experience and technique—like the KunJa of the Orient.

We can divide the world today into three parts: The material, the moral and the ideal. The martial artist's aim is to pursue absolute goodness in spirit—the "ideal."

Confucius said, "KunJa develops upward everyday, so he may reach through to the moral. A little man gropes downward each day so he may reach the material."

KunJa pursues cultivation of character and improvement of mind. He devotes himself to his work. Beyond that, he depends on nature and fate. Thus, he always has an imperturbable soul. He is the unity and harmony of man and nature.

The little man pursues comfortable living and achieves material goods.

Just as he attains this one good, he desires a new and better one. As he achieves more and more, he worries more and more about losing what he has gained. Thus he never achieves peace of mind.

Originally, human beings are equal at birth; their starting point is nearly identical. However, the KunJa "gentleman" and the little man pursue different and opposite paths. KunJa pursues the renowned world; the little man looks for profit. Finally, KunJa's path and that of the little man are far removed from each other.

Confucianism emphasizes the morals of human beings as a permanent fundamental principle.

The morals of humanity are based on social organization and establishment of proper do.

Establishment of this do requires certain values. Foremost between parent and child is love, between king and men is manner, between wife and husband is distinction, between old men and youth is respect, and between friends is faith.

We can still apply these values to today's society. For example: First, without parents, we do not exist. Parents are our roots, therefore we must have respect for them. Second, old people have experience and wisdom in life, thus they, too must be respected. This is one reason for the belt system in tae kwon do—respect for seniors. Third, not only must we have faith in friends, we must expand our faith to all human relations. Within material well-being, like a little man, we feel emptiness due to lack of faith.

In the Orient, the relationship between teacher and student is comparable to that of parent and child. Therefore, the father is the sun, the teacher is the moon. They have absolute position. The mind that respects his teacher is the foundation of education. If the student has no respect for the teacher, no trust in him, the teacher cannot influence his student's education. Those who are truly educated are always cautious, with a humble attitude.

Discipline and the relationship between student and teacher are important concepts deserving more consideration than they receive. A story within a story best points this out:

A long time ago, Bang Mong learned the art of the arrow from a man named Huyea. After learning all the techniques from Huyea, Bang Mong thought: "Who is better than I in the whole world? Only one!" He then killed his teacher Huyea, the teacher. About this, Mang Ja (ex-

ponent of Confucius) said that Huyea, the teacher, had made a tragic mistake.

He then had a story: In the old days, the Chung nation invaded the Wei nation, led by General Ja. The Wei nation counterattacked, led by General Yu. One day, Ja told his soldiers: "Today I am sick. I cannot use my arrow. If I err, I die. Who pursues us today?"

His men answered, "He is General Yu, sir."

Ja said, "Then I will live."

Confused, the soldiers said: "Sir, Yu is one of the best arrow men in Wei. How can you say that you will live?"

Ja said, "Yu learned his arrow techniques from Master Yong, and Yong learned from me. Yong is a man of good moral character. I believe that he would choose only a virtuous friend to teach the art of the arrow."

Later that day, Yu pursued and questioned Ja: "Sir, why do you not carry an arrow today?"

"Today I am sick, and I cannot hold an arrow," said Yu.

"Sir, I learned my arrow techniques from Yong, and I heard he learned from you. I cannot hurt the teacher who taught me the technique. But today, I am ordered by the King, whose orders I must obey."

He then picked up his bow and four arrows, breaking from each the tip, shot the four arrows into the air, and returned to camp.

In teaching the martial arts, we must teach the right person. If we teach a person who could kill his own teacher, the teacher is responsible also.

Martial arts must emphasize the spiritual side, KunJa and his ideals, in addition to technique.

If Columbus had not begun sailing toward the end of the earth, the discovery of America would have come much later. If J.F. Kennedy had not promoted the Apollo project, the moon would still remain a romantic object for poets and lovers.

Time must be taken to emphasize the great KunJa ideals and supreme virtues. The martial arts student must learn to use these ideals, to uphold and acquire virtues through action, and the martial arts teacher must show him how.

If he does not, the teacher creates the same problem for society as did the misguided teacher of the arrow, Huyea. To maintain the balance of nature, the power of tae kwon do action must be wielded by students with KunJa as their ideal (i.e., wisdom, human heartedness and courage).

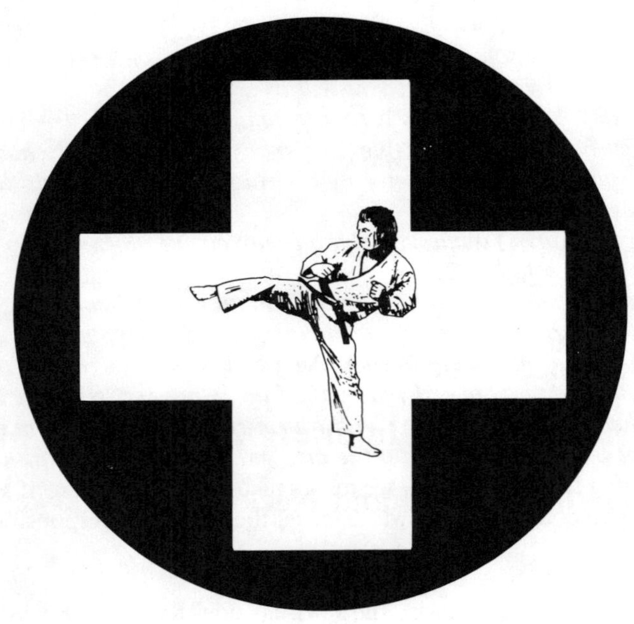

The treatments and activities suggested in this book have been developed by the author from his experience in the practice of medicine. However, every sports injury, and the reaction of the injured individual, is unique, and, therefore, the treatment or activity which is appropriate in most cases of a particular injury may be inappropriate in others. Accordingly, the treatments and activities described in this book may be inadvisable in certain instances.

CONTENTS

Introduction

A very important item of consideration in first-aid is often overlooked. That is, it is common to forget about the playing field or practice area as a potential source of injury. It is very important that the dojo be free of potential hazards to the student. Some dojo have folding chairs scattered about the sides of the room, barbells left lying at one end of the workout area, or a construction project left without a protective barrier. Each of these instances can lead to some type of injury if not considered as a potential hazard. The instructor and/or gym owner must always keep safety for his student uppermost in mind when preparing a workout area.

Here is a basic checklist to keep in mind:
1. The surface should be open and clear of obstacles.
2. The floors should be smooth, even and clean.
3. There should be adequate illumination of the training area.
4. There should be adequate ventilation.
5. All furnishings and maintenance equipment should be removed from the training area.
6. There should be separate areas for workout equipment such as weight training sets, universal gyms, etc.
7. The office area should be adjacent to the training area and equipped with nonbreakable glass or an open area for continuous observation of the whole dojo area.
8. A first-aid kit with adequate supplies should always be handy and accessible for immediate use (see chapter one).
9. There should be adequate floor space per student.

If these basic rules are observed the instructor has already taken a giant step toward a safer gym environment.

It is not my purpose to advise on the building design of a dojo. From a medical standpoint, however, I do want the instructor to be aware of a safe working space between students in both karate-type and judo-type activities. When a class is working together on kick exercises, it is important that each student have adequate room between him and his classmates during the exercise. Hand techniques can be done with less space between students.

For kicking movements, especially in lower belt classes, I would recommend a six-foot space on all sides of the student as a minimum space. That way, there will be a 12-foot-square available for most major moves except jump techniques. This will eliminate accidental collisions during floor exercises. An experienced instructor can accurately gauge the space needed between students for the various exercises used during class.

There is one more item that is offered as a suggestion to gym owners. It is not directly related to first-aid, and so I add it on the end of this introduction:

Gym owners would be wise to investigate the availability of a medical insurance program that would cover injury in the practice setting, tournament injuries, and possible coverage during travel to and from martial arts events for sponsored teams. At this point in time, there is some discussion of offering a relatively inexpensive medical insurance program through the AAU. I am sure that other companies will soon realize that there is a need and a market for insurance coverage in martial arts. Instructors and gym owners should keep their eyes open for further developments in this area. It is the sort of protection that could keep the business end of the gym solvent.

The martial arts business is becoming a multimillion dollar enterprise in the United States. It is time for the leaders and owners to realize that they cannot rely forever on the goodwill of all students (and their parents) who will pass through the training halls. ■

CHAPTER 1
BASIC FIRST AID

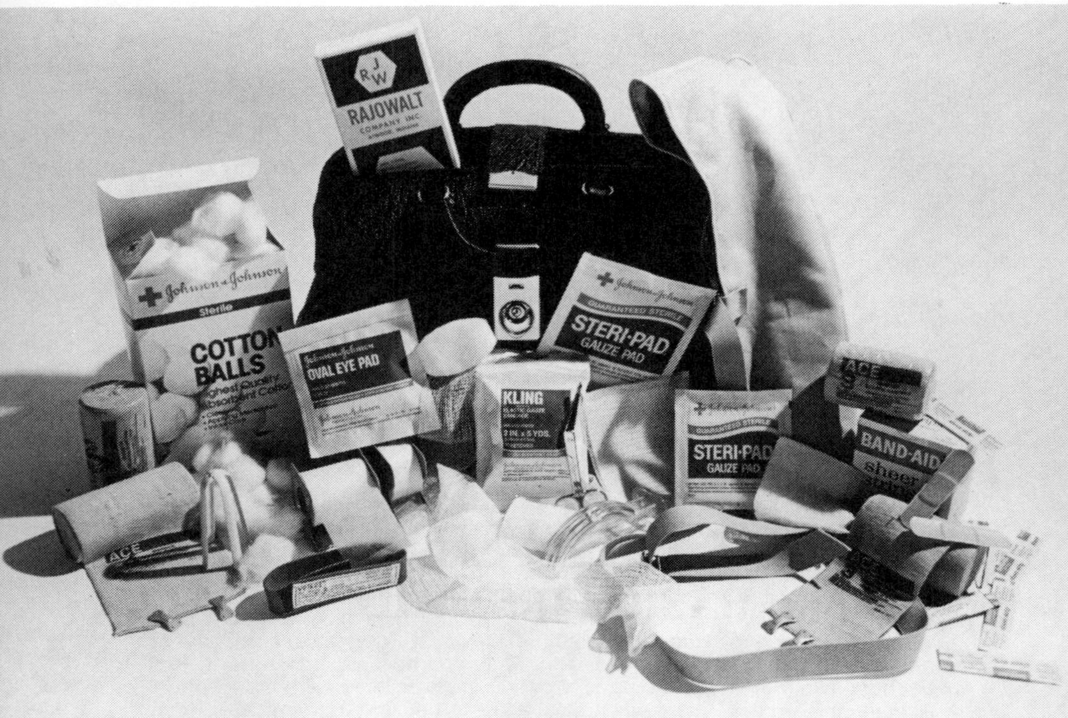

The basic first-aid kit should be large enough to hold the supplies listed on page 15. It should be unlocked and available during class time. All supplies in the bag should be clearly marked on the outside of their packages, and used items should be replaced immediately to avoid running out.

THE FIRST-AID KIT

Being prepared is the first step in being able to adequately handle emergency situations when they occur. That is why each martial arts school should be equipped with a basic medical first-aid kit to handle minor injuries, and for more serious injuries there should be a list with the telephone numbers of nearby emergency centers and ambulance services posted in a convenient place. The emergency numbers could also be taped on the medical kit.

The kit should be large enough to hold the supplies listed below. It is not necessary to buy an expensive doctor's bag. A well-built, small, square carrying case, or even a large fishing-tackle box, would be an adequate container. It should be unlocked and available during class time. All supplies or medicines should be clearly marked on the outside of their containers. Used items should be replaced immediately to avoid running out when needed.

Here is a list of recommended supplies:

1. Gauze bandages (sterile) cut in 2"x2" and 4"x4" squares.
2. Gauze rolls 2" wide, (one box of 12) or Kling rolls 2" wide.
3. White porous tape in 1" and 2" rolls (six each).
4. A small package of cotton balls.
5. Elastic bandages, 3" or 4" wide.
6. Oval eye bandages.
7. Band-Aids of assorted sizes.
8. One pair of bandage scissors (has blunt ends and is designed to remove dressings without injuring skin).
9. Bayonet forceps (a small size can be purchased at a medical supply store).
10. Slings: A simple, adjustable sling; medium-sized. A triangular bandage can be substituted for the sling, but it requires being folded into a triangular shape and then being tied around the neck.
11. Splints: These can be commercially purchased or simple wood boards 4" wide and 12" long can be cut out of ¼" plywood. These should be wrapped with cloth or tape to avoid getting splinters. In a pinch, layers of cardboard or newspapers can be formed into a splint for temporary use. Finger splints can be purchased in assorted sizes from a drug or medical supply store. Aluminum-foam splints are very useful and can be cut into lengths and bent to form as needed.
12. A rubber tournaquet: 1" or 2" wide. A wide leather belt can also be used.
13. A plastic oral airway tube—a small and a medium size.
14. A small pocket flashlight.
15. A small refrigerator for ice supply. Waxed cups can be filled with water and placed in a freezer pack to make ice cups. These are very handy for immediate direct application to a bruise or a hematoma (both are explained later in this chapter). Ice cubes should also be available to put in a plastic bag.
16. Medium-sized plastic bags, used to apply ice to wounds.
17. A plastic container (like a dishpan) used to hold water for immersing a foot, ankle, hand or elbow injury.
18. An antibiotic ointment (for example, Mycitracin Ointment, which is non-prescription).
19. Phisoderm liquid soap, for washing skin wounds.
20. Isopropyl alcohol, for use as an antiseptic.

This is only a suggested list which would serve for most common minor injury problems that can occur. Such optional items as an inflatable splint for upper and lower extremities are really not necessary.

GENERAL FIRST-AID CONSIDERATIONS

There are some basic principles to be learned that will aid the instructor and student in handling injuries that commonly occur in a gym or dojo.

Blisters

Anyone who has taken karate instruction will remember his or her first blister. They seem to be part of the training process for the beginner with tender, uncalloused skin on the feet. Blisters occur commonly in karate due to the fact that most gyms have a hardwood finish, and workout sessions are always in bare feet. The blister is a result of friction and pressure on the skin which is not toughened by previous conditioning.

The initial care of a blister is very important to prevent infection at the site of the blister. When infection occurs, treating and healing a blister becomes much more difficult.

Treatment of the blister is directed toward thorough cleansing of the area with soap and water followed by application of a Band-Aid or a small gauze dressing and tape. If the blister is partially torn open with a piece of skin remaining (which seems to always occur with blisters from karate activity) the injured area should be cleansed and completely dry before applying a wide Band-Aid with the blister flap laid flat over the open area to cover it. The Band-Aid should be applied smoothly with pressure over the flat area, and then a strip of tape should be laid over this. The tape strip should be wrapped all the way around the toe or foot to hold it in place during workouts. The sooner this can be done the less chance there is for infection. It is for this reason that the instructor should allow his students to attend to a blister as soon as it occurs rather than waiting until the end of a training session. Many times, if this treatment is followed, the flap will actually seal itself and heal over without a large open area left that usually heals slowly and painfully. Even if the flap does not seal over, it still provides a natural cover over the open area, and it promotes healing. If a blister becomes infected, the top should be "unroofed" with a sterile blade or knife, and then a sterile dressing should be applied.

Abrasions

A very common injury is an abrasion or floor burn. This is a superficial wound of the outer skin layer that has a raw, scraped look. The wound may bleed slightly or not at all. Usually the wound contains no debris since it occurs on a wood or tile floor. Occasionally, however, such an injury can occur outside while training, and then the abrasion may have dirt or grass embedded in the skin. The major concern here is to prevent infection. Basic treatment, therefore, is concerned with thoroughly cleansing the injured skin with soap and water, removing any dirt, grass or other foreign material. A soft-bristle brush or clean washcloth with a rough texture is ideal for this, and it is not particularly painful if it is done gently, rubbing in a circular motion.

After cleansing, the abrasion may be covered with sterile Vaseline or an antibiotic ointment (for example, Mycitracin ointment) and wrapped with a lightly-rolled gauze. This immediately reduces pain and sensitivity in the injured area, and it prevents further exposure to infection. The wound should be cleansed and dressed daily until it has healed. The main point to make is that abrasions should not be left untreated or ignored since they are an easy source of skin infection. Here the old adage, "an ounce of prevention is worth a pound of cure" is very appropriate.

Bruises

The next most common injury to be considered is a bruise, which occurs as the result of a punch or kick to the soft, non-boney areas on the body known as subcutaneous tissue (see illustration #2) which is located between the skin and muscle layers. Bleeding occurs easily in the subcutaneous area due to the looseness of the tissue and blood vessels. Following a hard blow to the subcutaneous tissue, bleeding occurs due to the rupturing of the small blood vessels in the fatty tissue. When this occurs, there is almost immediate swelling of the injured area followed by a bluish discoloration. Immediate application of ice and a compressive-type dressing (like an elastic wrap) following a bruise greatly reduces swelling, bleeding and pain. This

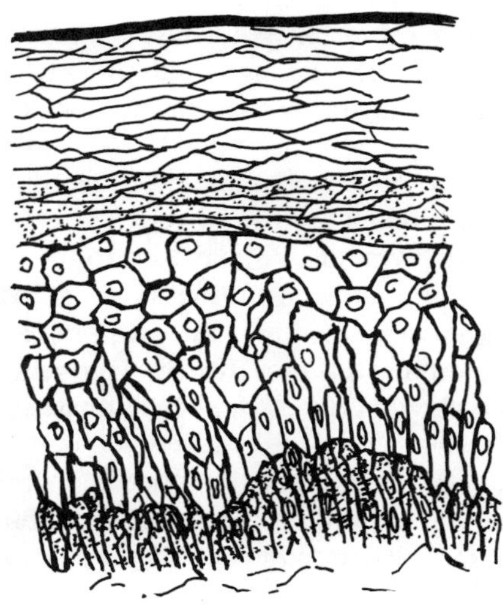

ILLUSTRATION #2

The subcutaneous tissue is the soft, non-boney area located between the skin and muscle layers. A hard blow to the body causes bleeding in this area, which results in a bruise. Applying ice and a compressive-type dressing (like an elastic wrap) will reduce swelling, bleeding and pain.

immediate-type first-aid will also reduce later stiffness and discomfort, and it will allow the student to return to training as soon as possible.

Ice application should be continued for at least 72 hours, or until the swelling goes down. After that, hot soaks or packs to the injured area will help the healing process. Larger, more painful bruises should be protected with a foam or rubber pad during sparring sessions to prevent further injury until healing is complete.

Very forceful blows can also cause injury to the muscle layer under the subcutaneous tissue. This may cause muscle fiber to rupture with immediate swelling and pain due to bleeding between the muscle fibers. The so-called "charley horse" is a rupture of the large thigh muscle (the quadricep), and it can occur from a strong blow or violent contraction of the muscle itself. Treatment again consists of applying ice immediately and then wrapping the injured area. Ice should be applied for at least 20 minutes at a time, two or three times per day depending on the severity of the injury. The injury should be rested, and activity should be reduced until swelling, pain and stiffness have decreased. Attempts to work out this type of injury will cause increased bleeding, among other complications. This, in turn, will cause the injured muscle to lose its ability to stretch and extend in a normal manner. When that occurs, the muscle is prone to easy re-injury and further loss of function.

Hematomas

Hematoma formation is a common injury in athletics involving physical contact. In karate, it results from a blow or kick to a soft part. A hematoma is a collection of blood in an area near an injury. Bleeding from the injured tissue collects in one space pushing other tissue away, forming a pocket of blood (see illustration #3).

Treating a hematoma should be aimed at stopping any more bleeding and then absorbing or removing the blood that has already collected around the injured area. Immediately applying pressure and ice to the injured area will help stop further bleeding and reduce the swelling. An elastic wrap applied with an ice pack incorporated into the wrapping accomplishes both purposes. (Large hematomas are best treated by puncturing the wound with a needle, but that should only be done by a physician under strictly sterile conditions.)

After pressure and ice have been applied, or after the blood has been removed by a physician, the hematoma site should be protected from further injury until healing is complete. Discoloration of the skin may be extensive following hematoma injury, but this does not indicate a more serious problem. It really is of little or no consequence, despite the discolored appearance.

ILLUSTRATION #3

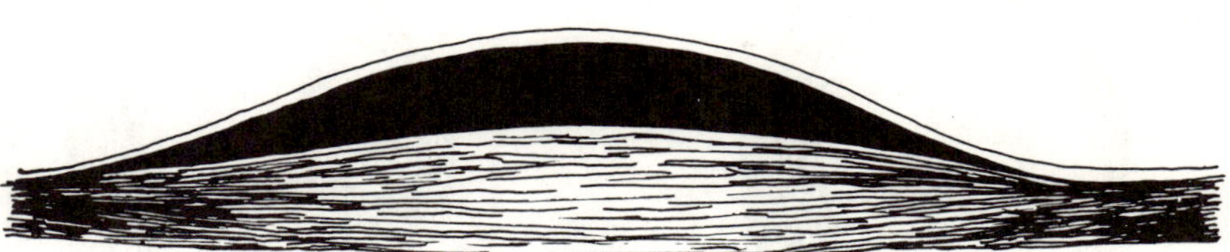

A hematoma is a pocket of blood which collects in tissue beneath the skin after a hard blow. Ice and an elastic wrap should be applied to the area in order to stop bleeding and reduce swelling. If the hematoma is large enough, a physician sometimes needs to be consulted to remove the blood.

Strains

Strains are injuries which occur in areas where muscles and tendons connect. (Muscles are attached to bone by tendons.) A strain results from overstretching, overloading or overusing a muscle or its tendon. It must be remembered that a muscle and its tendon operate as a single unit, and that injury to either part affects the other. A mild strain involves a simple tear of the muscle fibers. A severe strain involves a complete tear of the tendon from its boney attachment, and it results in a complete loss of function of the muscle-tendon group. Most injuries occuring in the martial arts are mild-to-moderate in nature. Completely tearing the tendon away from its boney attachment is rare.

Strains occur as a result of a sudden extreme force being applied to the muscle-tendon group. When the force that is applied to the muscle and tendon is greater than the area's ability to handle the load, a strain results. This is usually recognized by immediate pain in the muscle or tendon. Feeling around the injured area will reveal tenderness, and later there may be swelling and a sensation of stiffness of the area when motion is attempted.

Treatment of the mild-to-moderate degree of injury is directed toward protecting the muscle and tendon from further injury until healing is complete. Immediate treatment should include ice packs to the injured area followed by a compressive wrap with an elastic-type bandage. The injured part should be rested to protect it from further injury. Forceful, quick contractions of the injured muscle must be avoided until pain and swelling

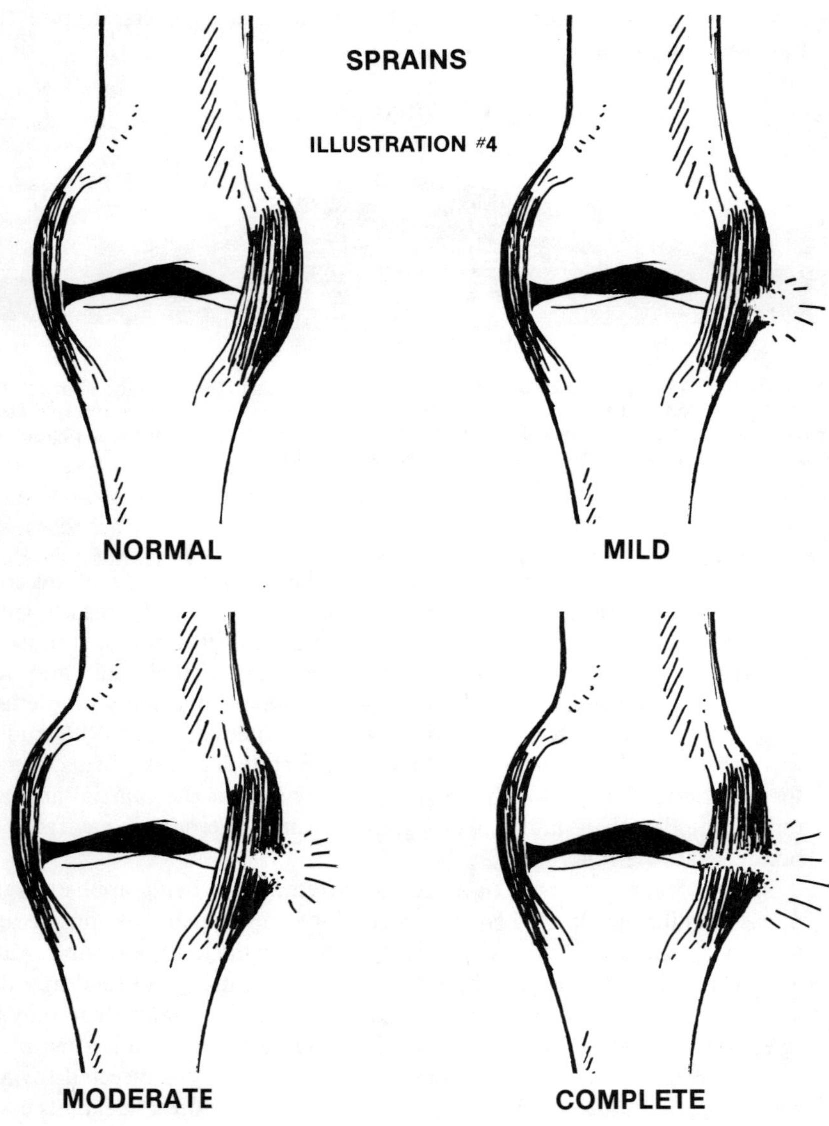

Ligaments are designed to hold two boney areas together at the joints. A mild sprain occurs when a small portion of the ligaments are torn away from a bone. A moderate sprain involves tearing up to half of the ligaments at a particular site. A severe sprain is a complete tearing of the ligaments.

subside. Daily stretching and slow contraction of the injured part along with ice application will speed recovery and maintain function. Premature return to full activity before healing is complete will result in a permanent, chronic injury to the muscle-tendon group, and it may impair the martial artist for life.

A severe strain is a rupture of the muscle and tendon from its attachment. This is a severely crippling and disabling injury, and it requires special attention by a physician trained in treating these types of injuries. Surgical repair will be necessary in most cases.

Sprains

A sprain is an injury to the ligament structure. The degree of the sprain depends on the amount of damage to the ligament and its attachment. Ligaments are designed to hold two boney areas together at the joints. The function of the ligament is to prevent excessive motion of the joint. A mild sprain involves a small portion of the ligament with only minimal tearing of the fibers. A moderate sprain involves up to half of the ligament fibers

ILLUSTRATION #5

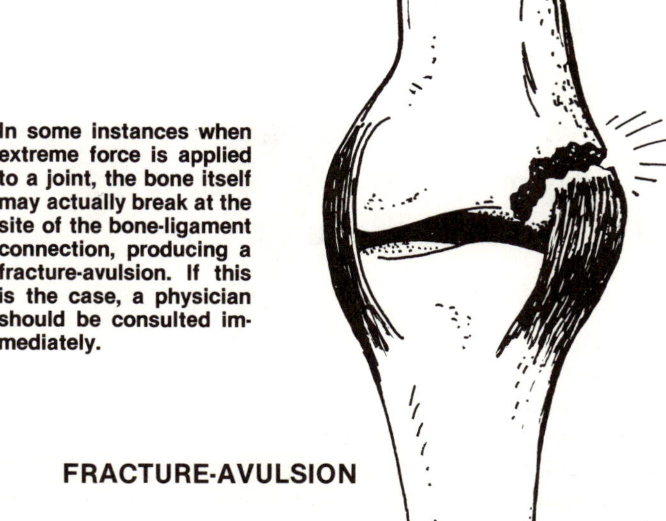

In some instances when extreme force is applied to a joint, the bone itself may actually break at the site of the bone-ligament connection, producing a fracture-avulsion. If this is the case, a physician should be consulted immediately.

FRACTURE-AVULSION

being torn. A severe sprain involves a complete tear of the ligament. (See illustration #4.)

The treatment of sprains depends upon the degree of the injury. Simple, mild sprains which involve only a small portion of the ligament require relieving symptoms only. This is best done by applying ice to the injured site. Activity can usually be continued without restrictions. A supportive elastic wrap is also helpful.

Moderate sprains are immediately painful and accompanied by swelling and some disability in moving the joint. Because the ligament is still at least 50 percent intact, there is no instability to the joint. The treatment of a moderate sprain is a much more serious proposition. The healing of a ligament is slow and requires six to eight weeks for complete recovery. (This is as long as the time required for a broken bone to heal.) Because of this time factor, the partially torn ligament must be protected by wrapping or strapping. Complete immobilization with a plastic cylinder is probably the best treatment of a moderate sprain, and it prevents further injury until healing is complete.

A severe sprain means a complete tear of the ligament, and it results in the loss of stability of the joint it is joined to. Treatment of this injury usually requires surgically repairing the torn ligament ends. Some cases may be treated with a cylindrical plaster cast, but most surgeons today are more aggressive and prefer surgery to restore the torn ligament.

When treating all soft-tissue and muscle/bone injuries, a quick and easy method to use is what is known as the *ICE* method:

$$I \; = \; \text{Ice on the injured part}$$
$$C \; = \; \text{Compression of the injured part}$$
$$E \; = \; \text{Elevation of the injured part}$$

The letter *R* could also be added, which stands for rest of the injured part in the early phase. So remember the letters *ICER* and apply them when these common injuries are encountered.

Also, using heat on acute muscle, tendon or ligament injuries is very bad during the first 72 hours. It will just cause increased swelling and make the injury worse. So instead, ice the injury first (during the first 72 hours), then add heat later after that three-day period.

CARDIO-PULMONARY RESUSCITATION

It is fundamental that all martial arts instructors and students have a working knowledge of how to use cardio-pulmonary resuscitation (CPR). Thousands of lives have been saved by non-medically trained people who have used this technique. To be able to resuscitate an unconscious person and prevent a needless death is a most valuable and rewarding knowledge to possess. The chances of a serious or life-threatening accident or injury in the martial arts is rare; regardless, one must always be prepared mentally with prior knowledge for the rare and unexpected event. It may only happen once in your lifetime, but it may mean the difference between life and death for someone, or even yourself.

Any person in an unconscious state who is not breathing has only about three minutes before permanent brain damage occurs. After four minutes, death is imminent, and even if the person is resuscitated, there is usually little chance of that person ever being normal again. Because of this, it is vitally important that everyone be acquainted with CPR.

Cardio-pulmonary resuscitation is based on the principle of restoring adequate circulation of the blood from the heart and adequate ventilation of the lungs. This is accomplished by combining external cardiac compression of the chest wall with mouth-to-mouth resuscitation. The procedure requires no special equipment in order for it to be performed. It does require a knowledge of the technique and when to use it. CPR must be started *at once* in any situation where breathing and a pulse are not detectable. You do not have time to go for help or ponder what to do. You must act immediately if you are to save a life. First, determine if the unconscious person is breathing. If he is breathing, you may assume that his heart is still functioning, because breathing always stops before the heart arrests. If there is no detectable breathing, check for a pulse. This can be done by feeling for a pulse in the carotid artery of the neck (see page 39). You can also place your ear over the upper-left side of the chest just to the inside of the nipple and listen for a heart beat. If there is a weak or absent pulse and no sign of breathing, begin immediate CPR.

In order to learn CPR effectively, think of it as an *ABC* process:

$$A \ = \ \text{Airway}$$
$$B \ = \ \text{Breathing}$$
$$C \ = \ \text{Circulation}$$

CARDIO-PULMONARY RESUSCITATION

1

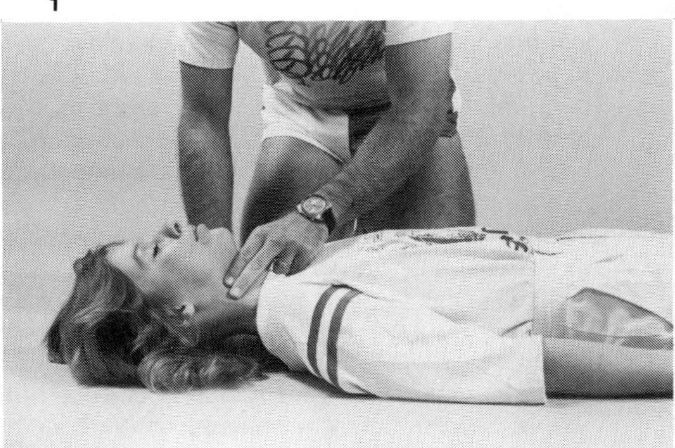

4

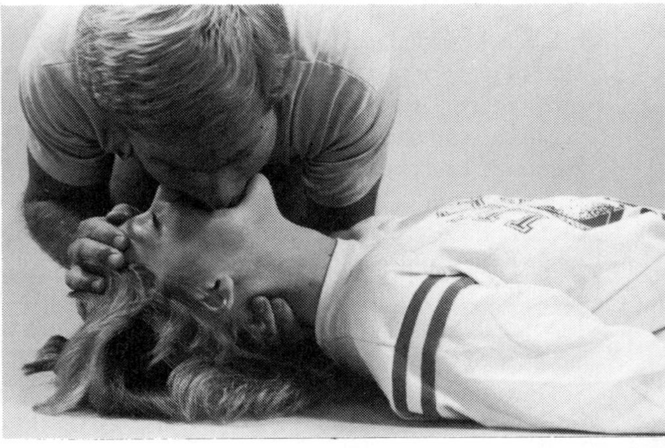

ILLUSTRATION # 6

The CPR process first involves checking the victim for a pulse, which is done by (1) placing two fingers over the carotid artery. Next, the victim's airway passage should be opened by (2) extending the head. The mouth (3) should be cleared of all debris to make breathing easier. If the victim is not breathing, mouth-to-mouth resuscitation (4) must be administered im-

2

3

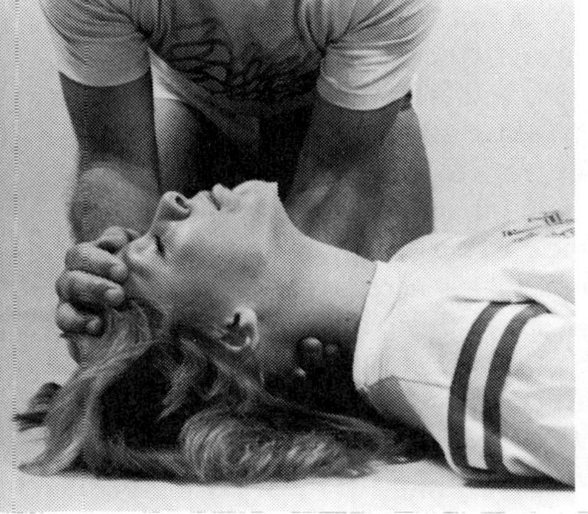 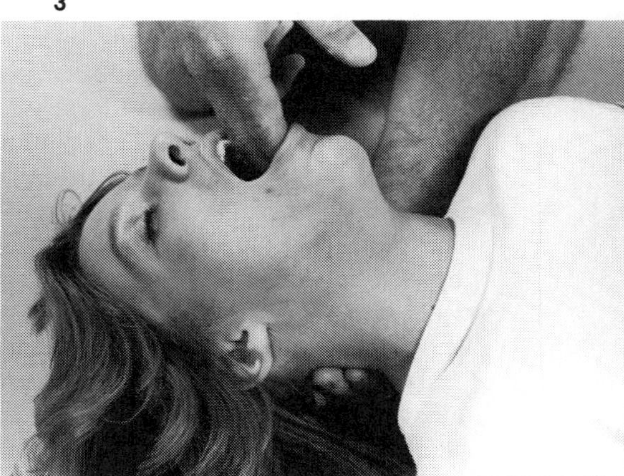

5

6

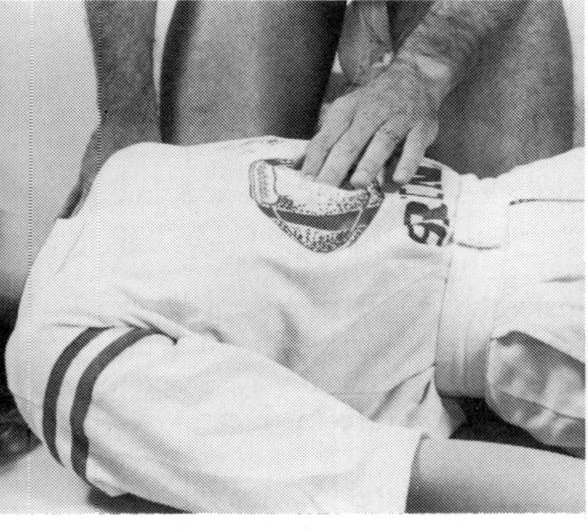

mediately. Administering 12 forceful breaths per minute, this maneuver will usually restore spontaneous breathing if the heart is beating effectively. If it is not, then cardiac massage must be administered. This is accomplished by (5) finding the lower end of the breastbone. Then (6) both hands are placed together over the victim's chest with the heel of one hand placed over the other hand, and all fingers elevated so they are not resting on the ribs. Press downward, then quickly lift your hands to their original position, allowing the chest to expand. This cycle should be repeated at the rate of 60 compressions per minute, or one per second.

Airway means opening the person's airway to provide adequate ventilation. This is accomplished in an unconscious person by extending the head.

When a person becomes unconscious, the floor of the mouth and tongue relax completely. This allows the tongue and muscles at the base of the tongue to fall back into the back of the throat causing an obstruction to the lungs. This is sometimes referred to as swallowing the tongue, which is a misnomer since the tongue certainly is not swallowed; instead, it is merely displaced by relaxation and gravity into the back of the throat. The head may be extended by lifting the neck with one hand and tilting the head back with the other. These two maneuvers lift the jaw and tongue, and they establish a straight, open airway from the oral cavity to the lungs.

Breathing is accomplished by artificially inflating the unconscious person's lungs. This is done by mouth-to-mouth resuscitation with the airway opened by extending the head. This is all that is necessary to replace oxygen into the lungs and bloodstream. Usually this maneuver will restore spontaneous breathing if the heart is beating effectively.

Circulation is restored by external cardiac massage after establishing an airway and inflating the lungs four to five times. When you cannot feel a pulse, the heart is either in cardiac arrest or beating weakly in an irregular, ineffective manner. When this has been determined, external cardiac compression should be started immediately.

Now, let's go through the details of the *ABC* approach. First, assume that you have an unconscious person lying on the floor, and that you cannot detect any breathing or pulse. Having done this, position the patient on his back. Always make sure that there is a firm surface under the person before beginning CPR.

Now begin mouth-to-mouth resuscitation. Remember, lift the neck and tilt the head back to open the oral airway. Next, open the person's mouth, place your mouth over his and make a tight seal with your lips. Blow into the person's airway strong enough to make the chest rise. Remove your mouth, turn your face toward the person's chest, and observe the chest fall inward and hear and feel the air being expelled from the airway. Begin a rhythmic mouth-to-mouth maneuver of about 12 forceful breaths per minute.

External cardiac compression is easily accomplished by placing the heel of one hand in the center of the chest over the lower end of the breastbone. The heel of the other hand is placed on top of the first hand. Elevate the fingers of both hands so they do not rest upon the ribs. With the hands in this position, press downward, using the weight of your upper body, and depress the sternum downward toward the backbone 1-1½ ". This external compression compresses the heart, which is between the sternum and the spine. The blood is then mechanically forced out of the heart into the body and lungs. After compressing the chest, quickly lift your hands to their original position, allowing the chest to expand and the heart to refill with blood. This cycle is repeated at the rate of 60 compressions per minute, or one per second.

The hand position should remain the same during relaxation as during the external compression. Your body should be positioned to the side of the person so that your hands are directly over the mid-section of the breastbone, and you should be kneeling if the person is on the floor.

CPR is most efficient when done by two people. One person extends the head and inflates the lungs at a rate of 12 times per minute while the other person begins external cardiac compression at a rate of 60 compressions per minute. In the event there is only one person available, then he must alternate external cardiac compression and mouth-to-mouth resuscitation by giving two breaths after each ten chest compressions.

It is recommended that all karate and judo instructors be familiar with and able to perform these maneuvers when required. The American Red Cross, as well as other various health departments and police agencies, offer this training throughout the year to interested parties. ■

CHAPTER 2
FACIAL INJURIES

MARTIAL ARTS INJURIES

Facial injuries are usually minor in the martial arts due to the fact that actual contact is not allowed in training, controlled sparring, or tournaments. However, sometimes a lack of control or poor refereeing will lead to heavy facial blows. Full-contact karate, which is becoming more popular, will result in more serious injuries. The use of regulation-type padded gloves, headgear and footpads can reduce most cuts from blows in full-contact karate, but they will not prevent more severe facial injuries. Regardless of the degree of control and accuracy possessed by the expert practitioner, there will always be accidental strikes to the face resulting in various degrees of injury. As in all forms of contact sports, a certain risk must be accepted by the participant. The risk can be reduced by proper training and instruction, good protective equipment, and above all, excellent refereeing, judging and medical supervision.

Facial cuts usually occur around the eyebrow, nasal area, cheekbones and lips, because most attacks are directed toward the center of the face by an attacker. Another factor is that most attacks are based on straight-type punches rather than roundhouse or hook-type blows. Kicking techniques are less likely to cause cuts; they are more likely to result in a bruise to the face and head from a well-placed strike. This is probably due to the fact that the foot has very few boney prominences and that most head attacks come from the side. Facial cuts are usually superficial, but they may bleed heavily due to the abundant blood supply to the face. Basic treatment should be directed toward controlling bleeding by direct pressure with a sterile or clean gauze dressing. Dabbing and wiping a cut only increases bleeding. Steady pressure to the cut for one or two minutes will control bleeding in most cases.

After controlling the bleeding, an instructor should then determine how deep the cut is. Gaping or jagged wounds with persistent bleeding indicates a deeper wound, and it will require careful surgical closure by a medically-trained person. Superficial skin wounds, which do not gape and respond to direct pressure, may be thoroughly cleansed with tap water and then covered with a Band-Aid or butterfly-type dressing (which is described in this chapter). It cannot be emphasized too much that thorough cleansing of the wound is very important. Infection of a simple cut is a much greater threat to the athlete than the skin injury itself. Simple cuts should be kept clean and covered until healing is complete in five to seven days. Any open wound which develops swelling with redness surrounding the opening is usually infected and should be evaluated by a physician.

After pulling the wound together with a butterfly bandage or Steristrips, cover the cut with sterile gauze and tape, making sure the wound edges are dry.

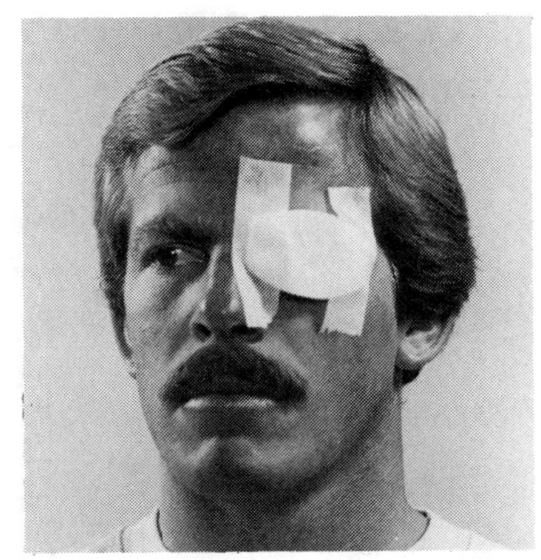

ILLUSTRATION #7

An eye pad should be worn following an injury to the eye to protect it from further injury.

EYE INJURIES

The boney structures around the eye provide a protective cage to the globe, especially against a blow from a large object. The smaller the surface area of the striking object, the more likely it is there will be an injury to the eye itself. Because of this, finger attacks to the eyes should never be done in practice or sparring because of the serious chance of permanent blinding or impairment of vision. It is strongly recommended that the instructor be aware of any student with an eye impairment. Any participant with a previous eye injury or decreased vision should be advised to wear protective eyeglasses for all attack exercises and sparring. The instructor should also be aware of all contact lens users. These students should either remove their contacts during practice, or if they are necessary in order to see, protective glasses should then be worn during class.

The most commonly encountered injury around the eye is probably a black eye, resulting from a direct blow. The first consideration with this type of injury is whether there has been any serious damage to the actual eye portion itself. Following a direct blow to the orbital region, the softer parts around the eye will immediately swell up and bleed. There is a simple examination procedure which can be used to determine if the eye has been injured; observe the lids for any cuts, and make sure both eyes move together normally. (If they don't move together, there may be a fracture to the boney area around the eye, and that would require immediate care by a physician.) After inspecting the lids and eye movement, check the globe itself to see if it is bleeding. Any blood in the eye that is not leaking in from an outside cut means there is a potential threat to the eye's vision, and that would require an immediate evaluation by a physician, preferably an ophthalmologist.

CHECKING EYE DAMAGE

ILLUSTRATION #8

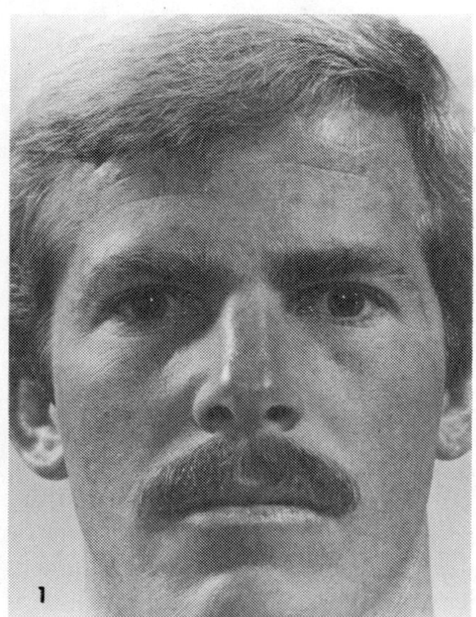

To determine how severely an eye has been injured, (1) first check the lids for any cuts. Then (2&3) have the victim look right then left to make sure both eyes move together normally. If they do not, there may be a fracture to the boney area around the eye, and that would require immediate care by a physician.

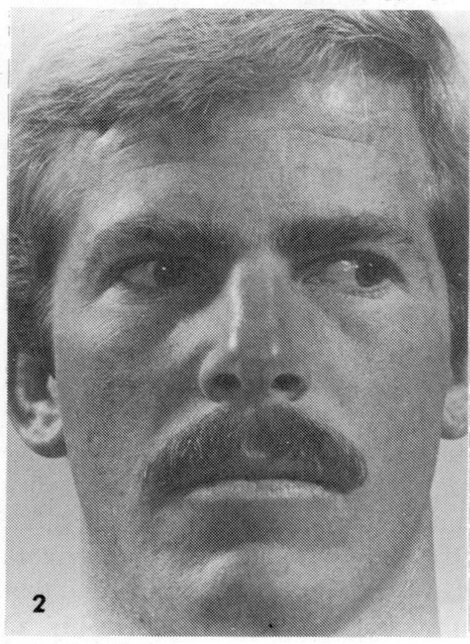

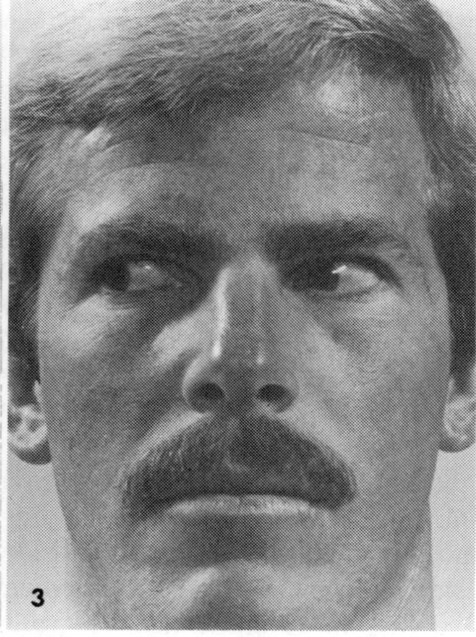

ILLUSTRATION #9

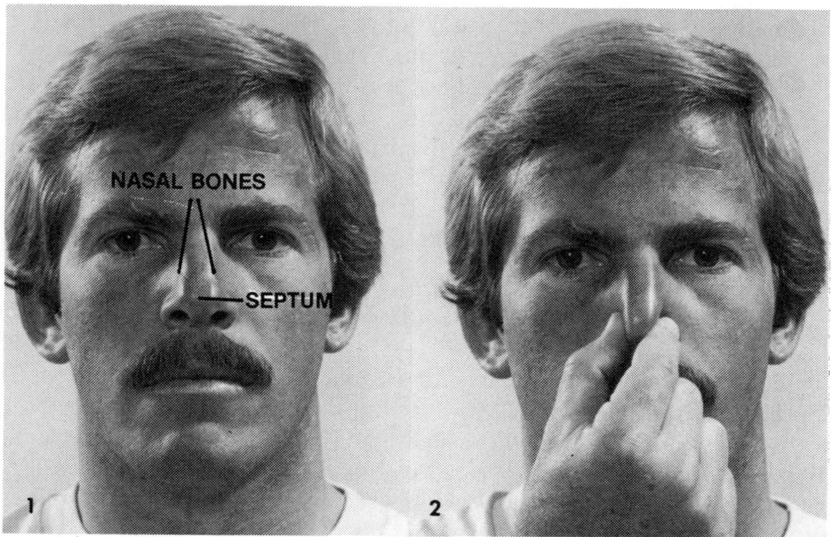

The most common nose injury, the nose bleed, is usually easily controlled by direct pressure with a cold cloth or ice pack over the side that is bleeding. Pinching the nostrils (2) is also an easy method for controlling such injuries. If a nasal fracture is suspected (if the nose is flattened, or the nose deviates to one side, or if bleeding persists, or if it is difficult to breath through one side), *gently* feel along the nasal bones and if there is a tender irregularity along the bridge, that usually indicates a fracture. The victim should then be taken immediately to a physician.

NASAL INJURIES

The nose is a common target for injury in the martial arts because of its central location on the face and the fact that it extends out from the face. Nose bruises are common and result from direct blows to the nasal area, usually during free sparring. A bruise may be recognized by minor swelling and tenderness. A careful inspection of the bridge of the nose will reveal any deformity or deviation. Immediately applying ice will decrease swelling and tenderness. This should be applied as an ice pack (crushed or cubed ice in a plastic bag) for 10 to 15 minutes, two or three times a day until the swelling has subsided.

Nose bleeds are also common. They are a result of injury to the inner lining of the nose, the septum or the nasal bones, or a combination of both. (See illustration #9.)

Nasal fractures should be suspected when there is an obvious deformity (flattening) or deviation of the nasal bones to one side, persistent bleeding or an obstruction of breathing through one or both sides of the nose. Gently, carefully feeling the nasal bones will sometimes reveal a tender irregularity along the bridge of the nose, which usually means it has been fractured. When this is suspected, the participant should be referred to his physician or an emergency room for further evaluation. Bleeding from the nose that cannot be controlled by external pressure will require internal nasal packing, and that should be done by trained medical personnel only.

EAR INJURIES

Ear injuries are less common in karate, but they are more likely in judo, especially during mat work. Most ear injuries are bruises resulting from the outside part of the ear being smashed against the bones of the skull. Immediate ice application followed by a pressure dressing will often prevent chronic scarring and the development of "cauliflower ears." Injuries to the ear which result in swelling and bleeding that cannot be controlled by ice and pressure should be evaluated by a physician to prevent permanent scarring and deformity of the ear.

An eardrum injury should be evaluated and treated by a physician as soon as is feasible in order to avoid permanent hearing loss. It results from a direct blow to the side of the head over the ear with an open or cupped hand. There will usually be immediate pain and a decrease in hearing, and the canal may bleed. It is important to avoid putting drops or other types of medication into the ear canal at this time, because it may cause infection in the middle ear. The injured person should also be told not to blow his nose, because it could cause further damage in the inner ear.

FACIAL FRACTURES

Facial fractures occur because of forceful blows from hand or foot attacks. Because it is a very serious injury, it is not within the boundaries of this handbook to describe proper treatment, but the instructor should at least be able to identify a facial fracture. The most likely fractures to occur will be around the cheekbones, the nose or the jaw. Cheekbone fractures should be suspected when there is swelling and pain which persists after a direct blow to the area. Gentle pressure with the thumb and finger over the injured area will reveal marked tenderness and increased pain. A jaw fracture should be suspected when the injured participant experiences pain when he clenches his teeth. He will also notice pain and swelling over the jaw bone itself.

Any suspected facial fracture should be sent to an emergency clinic for X-rays and further evaluation. Do not allow this person to continue further practice or sparring under these circumstances.

TONGUE INJURIES

Tongue injuries result from the tongue being crushed or cut between the teeth when a blow is struck to a partially opened jaw. It is wise to always instruct students to keep their teeth clenched and their jaw tensed during sparring to avoid this injury. Keeping the jaw tense by gently clenching the teeth also helps to reduce the effect of strikes to the lower face. If a participant does cut his tongue bleeding usually is a minor problem that can usually be controlled by direct pressure and ice application. If the cut goes completely through the tongue, it may require stitches. ■

CHAPTER 3
HEAD AND NECK INJURIES

MARTIAL ARTS INJURIES

Serious head injuries in the martial arts are rare, but they may become more common with the advent of full-contact karate. And despite the fact that most instructors and participants will never see or experience a serious head injury, it is very important to be familiar with recognizing and using basic first-aid in case it does occur.

Head injuries may vary from a mild disturbance in consciousness to a complete loss of consciousness or coma. Any participant who is dazed or rendered unconscious by a blow to the head requires careful observation to rule out a serious injury to the brain. Anytime a person loses consciousness as a result of a blow to the head or neck, the resulting injury must be considered potentially lethal. Never attempt to move or pull a person to his feet if he appears to be unconscious. Try to determine whether the injured person is breathing and has a pulse. If there is no sign of breathing or of a detectable pulse, immediately start cardio-pulmonary resuscitation (CPR described in chapter one).

If there are visable signs of a regular breathing pattern, do not attempt to move the person until you have determined whether there is a neck injury accompanying the head injury. If the person regains consciousness, do not allow him to sit up or move until you have evaluated the presence of a neck injury. Any complaint of pain in the neck, numbness or tingling to the upper extremities indicates a probable neck or spinal cord injury. *Do not move* this person without being acquainted with the proper precautions in moving a suspected spinal cord injury. This involves using continuous traction of the neck and transporting this type of injury on a firm backboard.

Any participant who has a period of unconsciousness after a blow to the head, even if only for a few seconds, should be evaluated by a physician before that person is allowed to return to regular practice. Any participant suspected of having an internal head injury should be taken to a medical center for further examination and treatment at once.

Other types of unconsciousness may occur from fainting. This can occur from a sharp blow to the abdomen, chest or throat. This type of injury occurs due to a stimulation of nerve centers involving abrupt blood pressure changes. In most of these cases, the person should be merely observed until they regain consciousness. It is important to make sure the injured person has an open airway and is breathing without difficulty. If you encounter a situation where the person is unconscious and not breathing, or if he appears to be strangling, you must act immediately: First check the mouth for the presence of any foreign material or dentures. If any foreign material is present, remove it immediately. Next, position the head and

ILLUSTRATION # 10

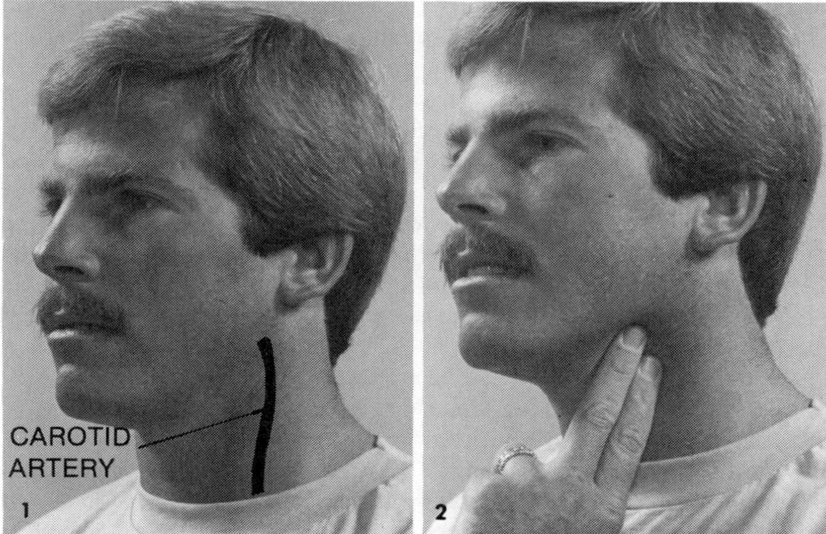

The carotid sinus nerve group, located (1) in the carotid artery detects changes in blood pressure. A pulse can easily be detected by placing two fingers (2) over the artery. Injuries to the area can cause a lower blood pressure, a slower pulse rate and a loss of consciousness. Treatment should be directed toward establishing an open airway for breathing, elevating the lower extremities 12″ to 18″, and performing CPR. (For CPR instructions, see page 23.)

neck in a hyperflexed position, which elevates the tongue and allows air to pass by the tongue into the lungs. This is usually all that is necessary to restore normal breathing in a person who has lost consciousness. In most cases, the person who has fainted will quickly regain normal consciousness without any serious consequences. Under these circumstances, when this occurs, it is best to excuse the participant from further practice for that session. CPR should be instituted in all cases where spontaneous breathing doesn't occur after opening the airway.

CAROTID SINUS INJURIES

Carotid sinus injuries are rare in all contact sports, but they can occur in the martial arts if the person receives a blow or pressure hold to the neck. The carotid sinus is a group of nerves located in the wall of the internal carotid artery (see illustration #10). These nerves are designed to detect blood pressure changes in the internal carotid artery and respond to these changes. Stimulation of these nerves can occur by pressure over the artery or by a direct blow to the side of the neck where the artery lies. The artery can be located by placing your finger just below the angle of the jaw and the sternomastoid muscle of the neck.

Injuries to the carotid sinus nerve group results in the lowering of blood pressure, slowing of pulse and a possible loss of consciousness. Persistent pressure to this area can lead to cardiac arrest. Treatment should be directed toward checking and establishing an open airway for breathing. Elevate the lower extremities 12″ to 18″ after placing the injured person on his back and performing CPR if no recognizable pulse or breathing pattern are present.

NECK INJURIES

Most neck injuries in the martial arts are of minor consequence, and they are usually either a strain or a sprain. Serious neck injuries, like head injuries, are rare. But when they do occur, a serious neck injury can represent the most serious threat to life and possible permanent disability to a martial arts participant. It is not within the scope of this book to give detailed treatment of neck injuries. It is important, however, for an instructor to be aware of the possibility and consequences of a serious neck injury.

The cervical spine is designed to provide a stable support for the head and yet supply a flexible arrangement which allows the head a wide range of motion. It is also designed to act as a unit to transmit major nerve groups from the brain to the rest of the body. Such an arrangement is an almost impossible combination to design and build from an engineering standpoint.

Neck injuries must be carefully handled and evaluated at the time of the immediate injury. Whenever a martial arts participant appears to have sustained a neck injury, it should always be considered a serious injury until further evaluation has been carried out. *Never* allow a person with a possible serious neck injury to sit up or stand up or move the head around until the injury has been carefully evaluated. While evaluating a head injury, always consider the possibility of an accompanying neck injury. Above all, do not be in a hurry to move the injured person so that the class may continue. To do so without proper evaluation and careful transportation may convert a moderate injury into permanent paralysis or even death. Move

ILLUSTRATION # 11

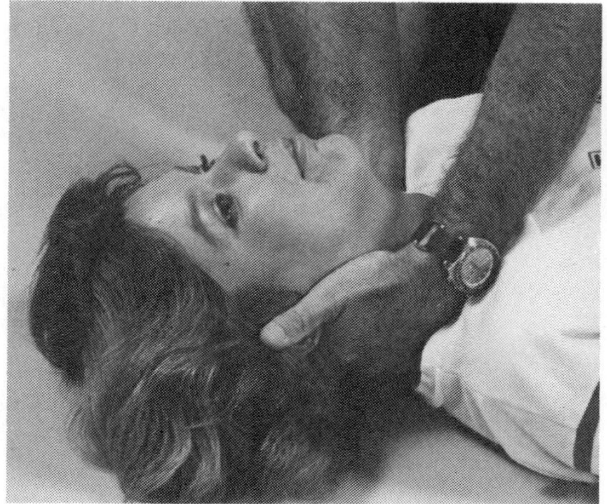

Neck injuries must be very carefully handled. The victim must remain on her back, and must not be allowed to move. It is always a good idea to cradle the person's head either by holding it in place, or by placing towels on either side of the head. Transportation by ambulance to a medical center should be immediate.

the class to the other end of the gym and begin a careful, unhurried evaluation of the injured person:

First tell the injured person to relax and not to move his head around if he is conscious. Ask if he has any pain and where the pain is. Ask if he has any numbness or tingling in any of his extremities. Next, ask him to slowly move his hands, arms, feet and legs. Severe pain in the neck or shoulders, weakness, numbness or tingling in any extremity, or inability to move the arms or legs indicates a possible severe neck injury.

If there is any question of a serious neck injury do not allow the person to sit up or stand up as this will cause a more severe injury if there is spinal cord damage present. Always support the head by gentle traction with both hands on the sides of the head, and roll the person onto his back. Following this, the injured person's head should be kept in a straight, neutral position by placing sandbags, towels, newspapers or pillows on each side of the head or by simply having someone gently hold their head in place. Transportation by ambulance to a medical center should be promptly instituted.

Always remember in cervical spine injuries, the injured person should be kept on his back. Never attempt to move a person with a serious neck injury in a face-down position. Always attempt to immobilize the head so it cannot move in any direction. This will require constant attention by the person giving first-aid. Any excess motion of the head on the shoulders in a severe neck injury may result in complete paralysis or death. ∎

CHAPTER 4
INJURIES OF THE SHOULDER AND UPPER EXTREMITIES

Shoulder injuries are relatively common in both karate and judo-type activities. Most of these injuries are mild, simple strains or sprains. However, there is an increased incidence of more serious injuries to the shoulder girdle when throwing techniques are involved. This occurs when the athlete is thrown on his shoulder or when the upper extremity is grasped and used as a fulcrum to throw an opponent.

The shoulder girdle is composed of several interconnected units which function together as one. An injury to one portion of the shoulder girdle affects the other shoulder components. Basically, the shoulder is composed of three parts, or components: 1) the joints; 2) the joints' accompanying ligaments; and 3) the muscle/tendon groups. The collarbone serves as a strut above the chest and sternum, and it keeps the upper arm from falling forward over the chest. The collarbone, along with the wing bone, suspends the upper arm from the shoulder girdle and provides the main ligament connections to the chest. The three main ligament connections are: 1) the inside end of the collarbone to the sternum; 2) the outside collarbone connection to the upper end of the wing bone; and 3) the upper arm to a concave-shaped portion of the wing bone (see illustration #12).

Each of these connections are provided with ligamentous structures binding bone to bone. The muscular units are made up of the muscles binding the thorax to the wing bone and the rotator cuff muscles of the shoulder.

Most strains of the shoulder involve the tendon attachments of the bicep muscles, and they result from exercise or the overload of these muscles from repeated punching or hand strikes. This will result in a tendonitis or bursitis of the shoulder. Tears or ruptures of the shoulder's muscles or tendons are rare in the conditioned athlete. They are more likely to occur in the novice or unconditioned person.

Pain with motion of the shoulder is the most common symptom of a shoulder strain. If there is pain, carefully feeling the muscle and tendon attachments will usually reveal a tender area. Treatment is basic and involves: 1) ice application; 2) rest of the injured area; and 3) supporting the arm with a sling and swath (see illustration #13). Ice should continue to be applied up to 72 hours after the injury occurs, 20 to 30 minutes at a time, three times a day. A sling and swath should be applied to provide rest and support of the injured area.

Following ice application for three days and rest with a sling, heat application and active exercises should be started. (The pendulum and Codman exercises outlined in Chapter 7 are helpful in increasing the shoulder's range of motion).

ILLUSTRATION # 12

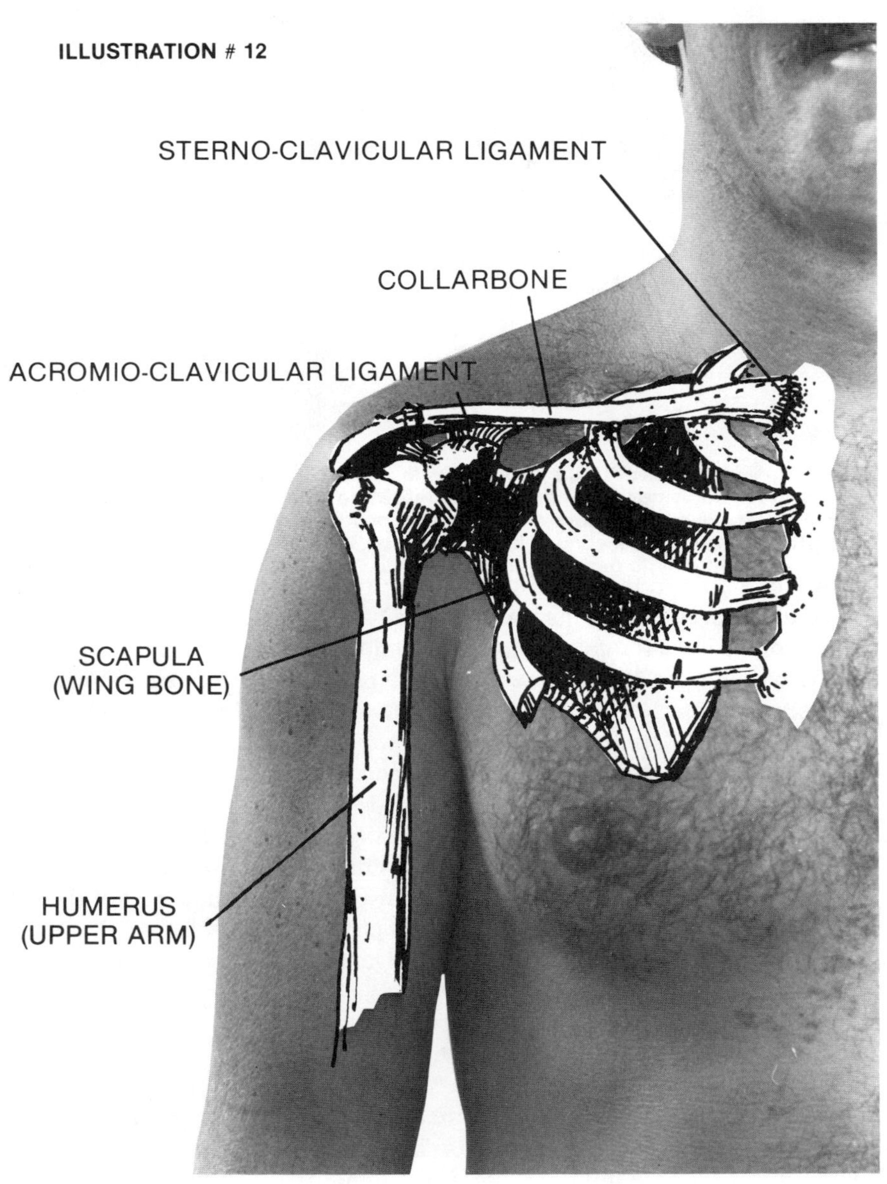

TREATING SHOULDER INJURIES   ILLUSTRATION # 13

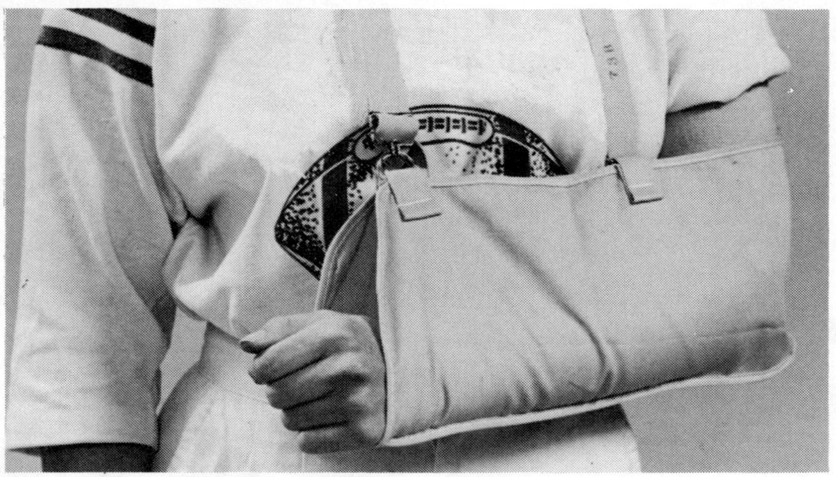

When a bone or ligament in the shoulder is injured, the best possible treatment for it includes applying ice to the injured area, 20 to 30 minutes at a time, three times a day for up to three days after the injury occurs; resting the shoulder; and supporting the arm with a sling to keep it inactive. Wrapping the arm in the sling with a swath (an elastic bandage) is also helpful.

Shoulder sprains in the martial arts usually involve the outside ligament connection between the collarbone and the wing bone. It occurs most commonly by falling or being thrown onto the point of the shoulder. It can also occur by falling on an outstretched arm or elbow. Most cases will involve only a mild stretching of the *acromio-clavicular* ligament (see illustration #12), which is recognizable by tenderness over the tip of the collarbone and a slight indentation just outside the tip of the collarbone. Treatment involves applying ice to the area, resting it with a sling, and sometimes padding it for a short period of time. If there is a more severe ligament injury to the area, there will be a raised deformity at the tip of the collarbone. This will require evaluation by a physician and X-rays to determine how severely the acromio-clavicular ligaments have been torn.

COLLARBONE INJURIES

Collarbone fractures are usually rare in martial arts activities. It is important, however, that the instructor or person rendering first-aid be aware of this possible injury. Some of the things that cause a collarbone fracture are: 1) a direct blow to the mid- or outer-third of the collarbone (some self-defense techniques include a knife-hand blow to the collarbone); and 2) a severe force sufficient enough to dislocate the acromio-clavicular joint which may fracture the collarbone instead. (This type of injury could result from any throwing techniques where the person is thrown on the point of the shoulder or on an outstretched hand.)

A collarbone fracture is usually easy to recognize. The most important symptom is severe pain located in the area along the front of the shoulder. There is increased pain with any motion of the upper extremity on the affected side. Gently feeling along the collarbone will reveal an extremely tender, swollen area at the site of the fracture.

While the treatment is not within the scope of this manual, the instructor should be able to recognize this injury and render first-aid. If the examiner suspects a fracture of the collarbone he should immobilize the shoulder girdle with a sling and apply an ice pack to the tender, swollen area. These two actions will offer a great deal of pain relief. Following this, arrangements should be made to transport the injured person to an emergency center for X-rays and definitive treatment.

Another possible injury that can occur in this same area is a sprain or dislocation of the *sterno-clavicular* ligaments. The sternoclavicular ligament is located on the inside end of the collarbone, and it joins the clavicular end to the upper sternum (see illustration #12). This is a rare and uncommon injury in the martial arts, and it is more likely to occur in judo or aikido throwing techniques than in karate-type activities. The classic features of this injury are pain and tenderness over the sternoclavicular joint and pain when you elevate your arm above your head.

Treatment of this injury only requires applying an ice pack, placing a sling on the affected side, and resting until the pain and swelling subside. It is advised that raising the arm over the head be avoided for two to three weeks until symptoms subside. Pain and disability lasting over this period of time should be examined by a physician trained in orthopedic injuries.

ELBOW INJURIES

Elbow injuries occur in the martial arts as a result of falling on the elbow, overextending the elbow joint while punching, or during throwing techniques. Another mode of injury not commonly seen in other sports is an elbow injury due to breaking techniques. These injuries result from direct force to the elbow during breaking.

Elbow bruises are a common injury, and treatment is simple unless there is an accompanying hematoma (see page 19).

There are several boney prominences around the elbow joint, and these are bruised by falling on the elbow, being struck on the elbow, or during breaking techniques. The skin and its fatty layer are easily bruised due to the thin layer over the boney structure. There just isn't much padding in this area. Following this type of injury, there will be tenderness over the point of the elbow with or without discoloration and swelling. Treatment consists of applying ice to the tender area and applying an elastic wrap from the wrist to above the elbow joint. The elbow should be at a right angle when applying the elastic wrap (see illustration #14).

Occasionally after bruising the point of the elbow, bursitis will develop. This involves the *olecranon bursa* which lies over the point of the elbow between the skin and the boney portion. This injury will cause a prominent "goose egg" swelling right at the point of the elbow. Bleeding usually occurs, plus there is usually an accumulation of fluid in the sac between the tendon and the bone. There will be tenderness over the swelling when pressure is applied, and the elbow will have a tight sensation when flexion is attempted. Swelling should be controlled with ice and an elastic bandage during the first 72 hours after the injury occurs. Persistent swelling and tenderness over the point of the elbow will require a physician's care to remove the fluid, although this is rarely necessary. Most bursal swelling responds to ice and a pressure bandage, and a soft rubber pad worn over the elbow may help prevent re-injury.

Hyperextension injuries can occur in martial arts activities from throwing techniques, pressure holds, and overextending the elbow with improper punching techniques. When the elbow is overextended, the front portion of the ligamentous capsule is overstretched, and the result is a sprain. When this occurs, there is immediate pain and swelling in the bend of the elbow. Attempts to straighten the elbow will increase the pain following the injury. Treatment should be undertaken immediately with ice applied to the front of the elbow joint. Following this, an elastic wrap should be applied (see illustration #14), and the arm should be placed in a sling. Ice should be applied two to three times per day during the first three days. After that, warm soaks or whirlpool baths are helpful.

Because ligamentous structures are involved, healing will usually require up to four weeks in order to regain full, pain-free motion. During the first few days following the injury, the elbow joint should be restricted and placed at rest in a sling. Once pain and swelling subside, motion of the elbow should be increased gradually. Painful motions should be avoided during this recovery phase.

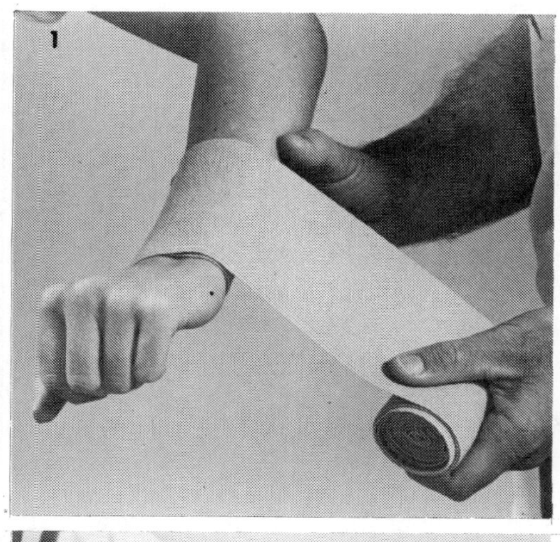

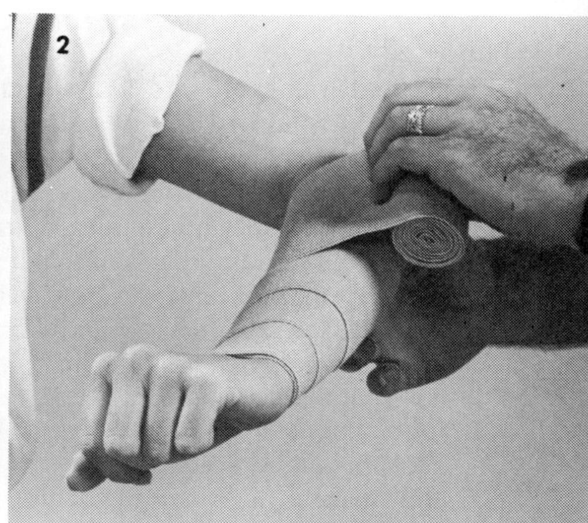

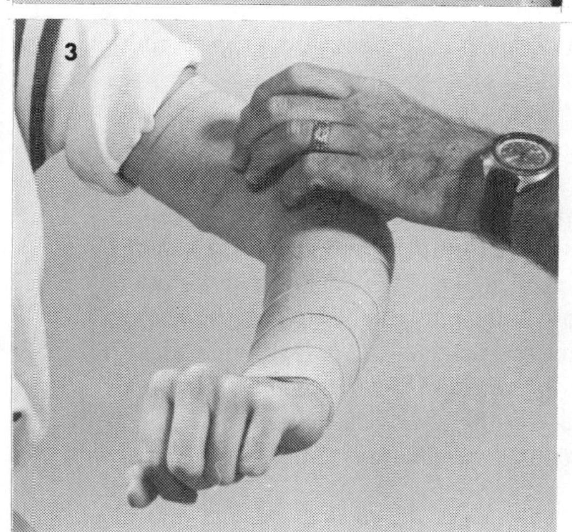

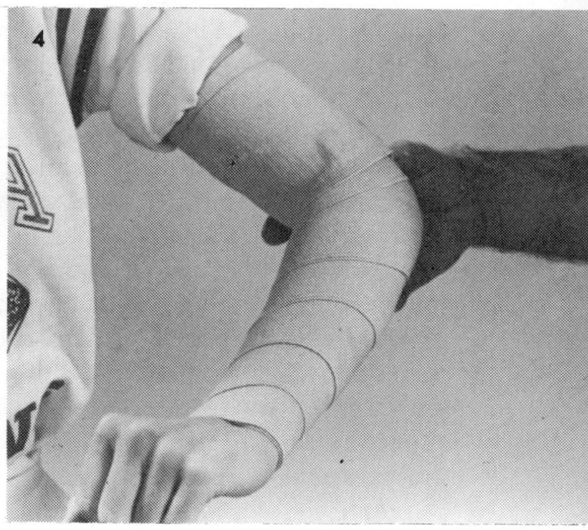

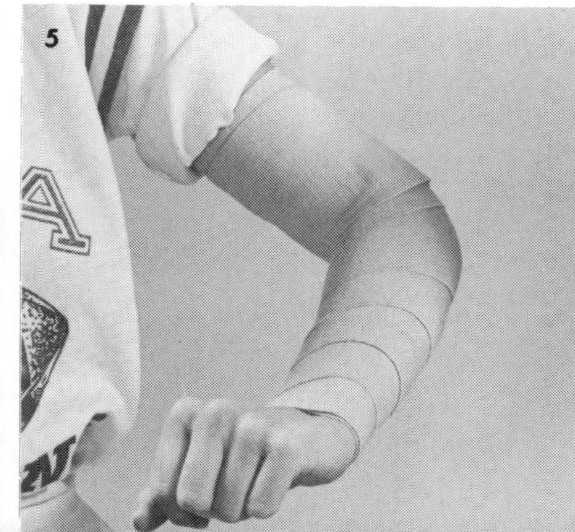

TREATING ELBOW INJURIES

Because there is not much padding over the elbow bones, they are rather easy to bruise. When an elbow is injured, ice should be applied to the tender area and (1-5) an elastic wrap should be carefully applied extending from the wrist up above the elbow joint. The elbow should be at a right angle when the bandage is applied.

ILLUSTRATION # 14

HAND INJURIES

Hand injuries are very common in karate-type forms of the martial arts. This occurs because the open hand and fist are used to strike the opponent or to block attacks.

Hand bruises are common and occur mostly at the knuckles when the fist strikes a boney part or a hard surface. Proper striking techniques (with the knuckle of the index and middle finger joints being the main point of contact) will help eliminate knuckle injuries. The knuckle joints of the ring and little finger are smaller and shorter and therefore more readily injured when they are used as the main point of contact. It is also important that the wrist remain straight and in a neutral position so that a straight line is formed between the elbow and the knuckle. Bending the wrist during the punching motion can cause a wrist injury as well as a knuckle injury. (It also weakens the power of the punch.)

Treatment of knuckle bruises consists of applying ice to the swollen joint area followed by a compression dressing with an elastic wrap. If there is persistent tenderness in the boney area and swelling after two or three days, the hand should be checked by a physician to make sure there is no fracture or tendon injury.

Thumb injuries usually involve the base of the thumb at the first *metacarpal-phalangeal* joint (see illustration #15). This injury is usually referred to as a "jammed thumb." A jammed thumb occurs when the thumb makes first contact during a hand strike. This occurs with circular-type hand attacks (hooks) or hand blocking movements where the thumb makes the first contact. It is important that instructors teach their students to execute hook-type hand strikes with the thumbs up and the elbow bent with contact being made on the hand and the knuckles. If the hook punch is performed with the palm down, it must be short, circular, and contact must occur on the large knuckle.

Treatment of a jammed or sprained thumb is directed toward reduction of swelling around the base of the thumb. This should be done immediately by applying ice or by immersing the hand in ice water. The thumb should be either splinted or placed in a thumb strapping with ½ " or 1 " tape. Splinting should continue until swelling and pain have subsided.

It is recommended that the jammed thumb be taped for several weeks after resumption of activity during practice.

Fractures of the metacarpal bone, or bones, can occur in karate-type activities such as contact sparring or breaking techniques. Most metacarpal fractures result from punching with a closed fist on a hard surface, such as

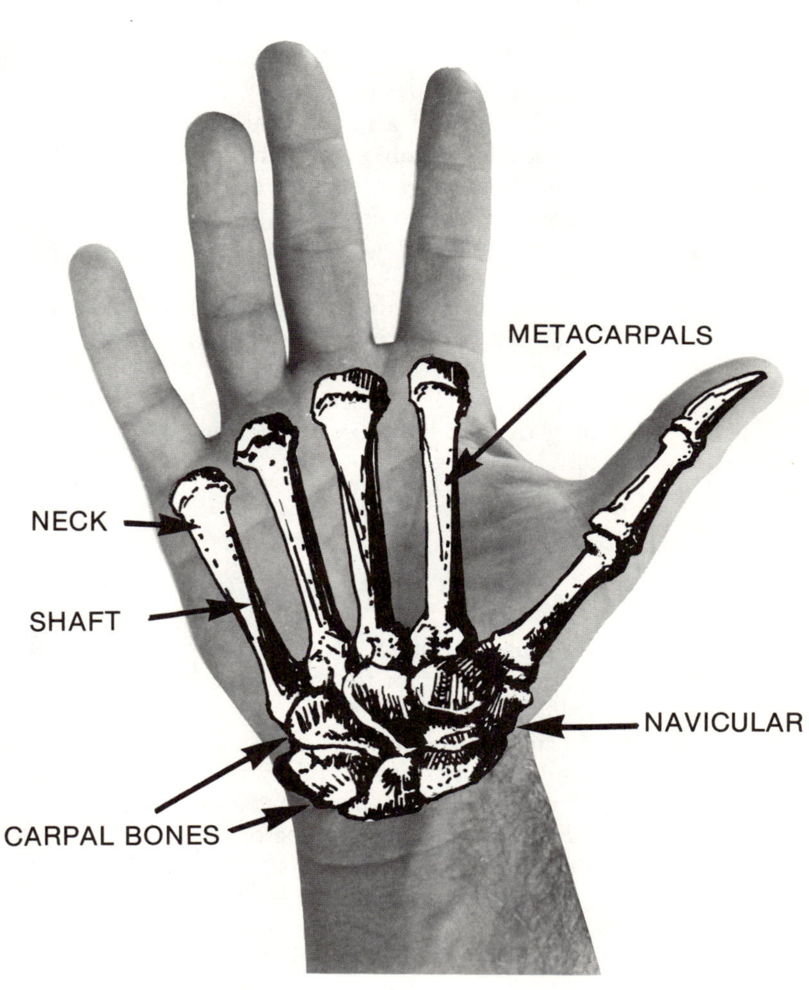

ILLUSTRATION # 15

THE WRIST

a boney prominence or wood or brick objects. Another manner of fracturing a metacarpal is striking an object with an open palm hand with great force. It is interesting to note that a fracture of the neck of the metacarpal can result from straight punching with the wrist slightly flexed (bent downward). A fracture of the shaft of the metacarpal results from a straight punch with the wrist slightly dorsiflexed, (i.e., slightly bent upward). For these reasons, it is important that the instructor makes sure that straight punches are delivered with a straight wrist.

Some of the characteristics of a fractured metacarpal bone are: 1) Immediate pain following striking an object with the fist or open hand; 2) Swelling over the back of the hand over the injured bone; 3) Pain on making a fist; 4) Pressure over the fracture site, which produces increased pain; 5) The finger of the afflicted metacarpal abnormally rotated as it extends outward from the palm.

If the examiner suspects a fracture of a metacarpal by the above criteria, he should stop the injured person from further activity. Immediate ice application over the swollen area of the hand should be instituted for 20 minutes, followed by application of an elastic wrap to prevent further swelling. After the basic first-aid the injured practitioner should consult his physician or go to an emergency facility for further treatment.

WRIST INJURIES

Wrist sprains are generally uncommon. Anytime one encounters a painful wrist after landing on the palm of the hand with the wrist bent, one should suspect a possible wrist bone fracture. The most common wrist bone injured in this type of injury is the *navicular* bone (see illustration #15) which lies on the thumb side of the wrist. Injury to the navicular causes pain in the wrist with any motion, and there may be some swelling in that area as well. And applying pressure over the anatomical "snuff box" will also increase pain at the fracture site. (The anatomical snuff box can be identified by opening your hand and extending your thumb outward away from the hand. When you do this you will note two tendons that stand out at the base of the thumb. As these two tendons enter the wrist, there is a depression between them. This is the so-called anatomical snuff box (see illustration #16).

Treatment of wrist bone fractures falls out of the scope of this manual. If the examiner suspects a fracture, however, the practitioner should stop

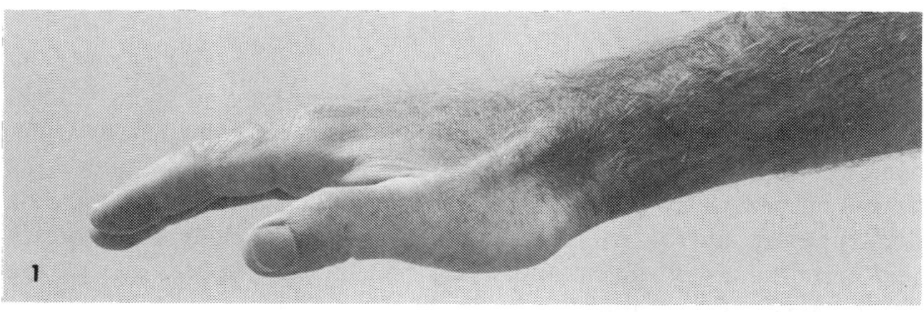

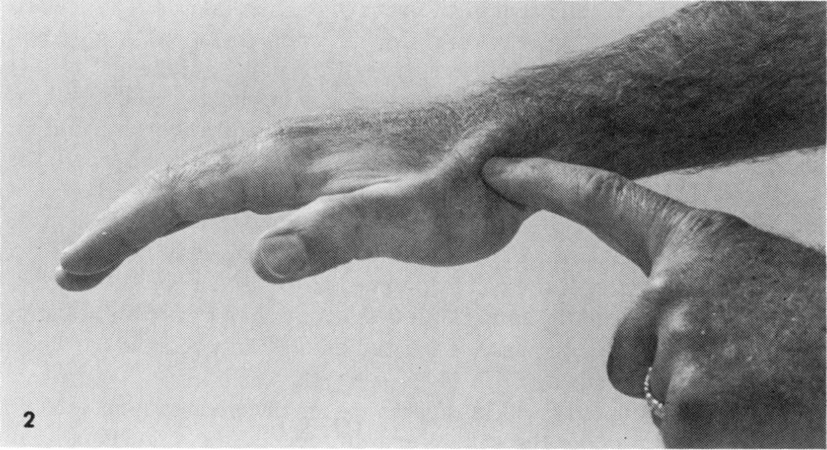

ILLUSTRATION # 16

The anatomical "snuff box" (so-called because it would appear to be a rather convenient place from which to inhale snuff) is located by opening your hand (1) and extending your thumb outward. As you do this, two tendons stand out at the base of the thumb. If a wrist injury occurs and a fracture is suspected, pressing in between those two tendons (2)—the "snuff box" area—will cause intense pain, meaning the wrist has in fact been fractured. A physician should be immediately consulted for X-rays and appropriate treatment.

practice activities, ice should be applied to the wrist as soon as possible after the injury, and a splint should be applied to immobilize wrist movement. A physician should then be consulted for X-rays and appropriate treatment. Appropriate diagnosis and early treatment will eliminate some rather disabling complications of the injured site. Many times a navicular fracture of the wrist will not show on an X-ray for up to ten days after the injury. An experienced physician will be aware of this, and will treat the injury with this in mind. The usual treatment consists of a plaster cast on the wrist and forearm for up to 12 weeks.

FINGER INJURIES

Finger injuries occur more commonly in karate-type activities than in judo or aikido because blocks and strikes are made with an open, or knife-hand technique. Injuries can be reduced using knife-hand techniques if the fingers are contracted tightly in side-to-side contact; the fingers should be slightly flexed, and the tendons of the hand should be held tense. A loosely held knife hand with fingers too straight and too far apart increases the likelihood of a finger injury.

Fingernail injuries can occur in all forms of the martial arts. They can be very painful, and it is an easy area for infection to set in. A common fingernail injury is the forceful separation of the nail from the nail bed. If the nail is only partially separated, it can usually be cleansed and then held in place with tape strips to avoid further ripping. It is important to treat this type of injury carefully to avoid having infection develop beneath the separated nail. Thorough cleansing with clean water and soap should be done immediately after the injury. A sterile Band-Aid should then be placed over the fingertip. Following this, tape strips may be applied to hold the nail in place. If the nail is loosened at the cuticle, or almost completely separated from the cuticle, it is best to consult a physician who may then trim a portion of the base of the nail or surgically remove the whole nail under local anesthesia.

Sometimes a fingertip will be stepped on or pinched, causing a blood blister to develop under the nail. When this occurs, the immediate treatment should consist of immersing the finger in ice water for 10-15 minutes. This will relieve pain and further swelling and bleeding under the nail in most cases. If enough blood accumulates under the nail, it is better to relieve the pressure by drilling a small hole through the nail after thoroughly cleansing the nail. A simple method of drilling a hole is to use a sterile #18-gauge needle or a #10 or #11 Bard Parker knife blade. The needle or knife blade is gently turned in a circular manner until the nail is perforated and blood oozes out from under the nail. After releasing the blood, the nail should be covered with a Band-Aid.

Puncture wounds of the hand can occur in karate-type activities when a fist strikes an opponent's tooth. This usually results in a human bite wound of the knuckle. *This is a very dangerous wound,* and it must always be considered a badly contaminated puncture or laceration. Do not treat this injury lightly or there could be very serious problems later from extensive wound infection. The human mouth and teeth harbor a great number of various kinds of bacteria. If these bacteria get into the hand after being

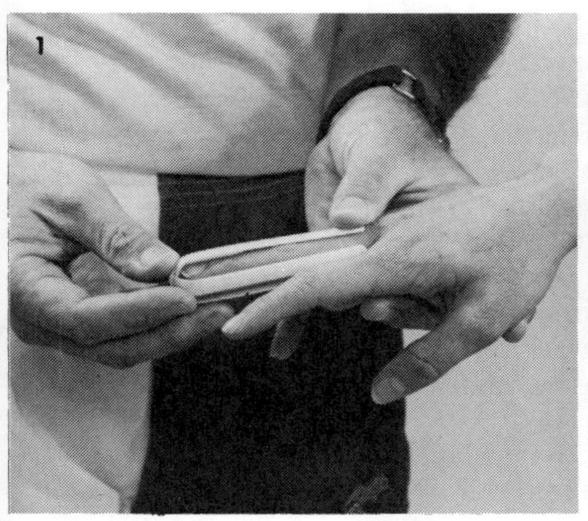

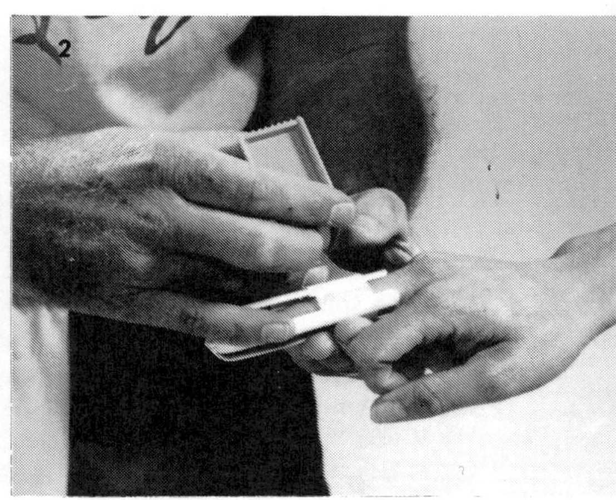

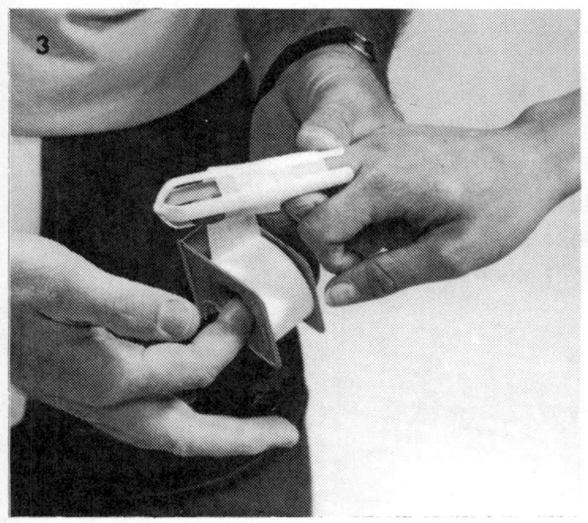

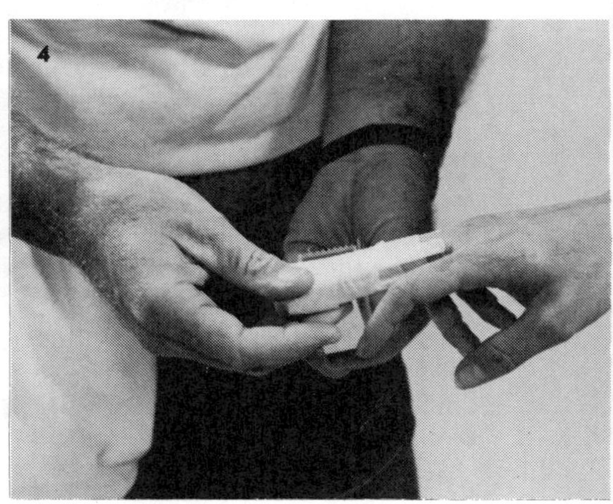

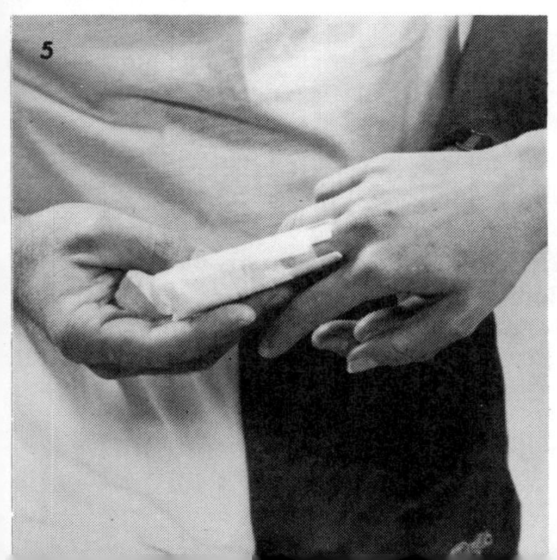

ILLUSTRATION # 17

TREATING FINGER INJURIES

If a finger has been sprained or if it has been dislocated, after pulling it back in the socket and icing it, the finger should be (1-5) splinted for up to four weeks. After that, the injured finger should be taped to its adjacent finger during practice for several more weeks until swelling, pain and stiffness are gone.

punctured by a tooth, a severe infection can result. Because of this, any wound resulting from a human bite must be thoroughly cleansed with a lot of water and soap. It is recommended that this type of wound be referred to a physician because of the high incidence of infections. A tetanus booster and antibiotics may be necessary.

Most finger injuries in the martial arts are sprains, and most finger sprains occur in the joint next to the tip of the finger. These sprains occur as a result of defensive blocks with an open hand against strong kicks. During sparring, beginning students should block with a closed fist until they have become adept at blocking movements. The finger is sprained when the joint which is nearest to the end of the finger tip is bent back too far, or when it is bent too far to the side.

When this finger joint is sprained, there is immediate pain followed by swelling. Feeling the joint will usually reveal where the tender area is. When the finger is bent back too far, there is tenderness over the top and bottom of the joint. And when the finger is bent too far to the side, the tender area will be in the sides of the joint. Treatment of a simple sprain consists of immediately applying ice or immersing the joint in ice water for 15 to 20 minutes. After that, the joint should be splinted with the finger slightly bent. Ice should be applied three times a day for 72 hours, and the splint should remain on the finger until pain and swelling have subsided, which may take up to three weeks. Once the joint has recovered, it is wise to tape the injured finger to its adjacent finger for at least a week following resumption of practice.

JOINT DISLOCATIONS

The joints of the finger are dislocated the same way they are sprained, but with greater force applied. When this occurs, the ligament capsule holding the joint intact is disrupted and the boney portion is forced out of its normal alignment. The injury is easily recognized by the obvious dislocation of a portion of the finger from its usual alignment, and it is always extremely painful.

Treatment should be directed toward immediately preventing swelling. This can usually be easily accomplished by grasping the dislocated finger with your hand, forcing the joint into hyperextension at the same time that traction is applied by pulling on the injured finger in a slow steady manner. Usually you will feel a definite click indicating the joint has been reduced to its normal alignment. Any dislocation that cannot be easily reduced should be referred to an emergency clinic as soon as possible. When the joint can be easily reduced after dislocation, the same treatment used for sprains should be followed, and the injured person should always consult his doctor for follow-up to make sure that a chip fracture has not occurred at the same time.

Following reduction of a simple dislocation, it is advised that the finger be splinted for up to four weeks. This allows the injured ligaments enough time to heal. It is also recommended that the injured finger be tape-strapped to its adjacent finger during practices for several more weeks until swelling, pain and stiffness are gone. ∎

CHAPTER 5
TRUNK INJURIES

The trunk is made up of the chest, abdomen and groin areas, and it comprises the major target area of the body in karate attacks if you exclude the head and neck. Most of the serious injuries to these areas have been eliminated by specially designed chest and abdominal padding used during practice sparring in the gym. In addition, groin injuries are less common because of groin cups.

CHEST INJURIES

Chest bruises occur from hand strikes or kicks to the front of the chest since this is a legal target area in tournament sparring. The injured participant will usually notice tenderness over the area that was struck. Occasionally the hand strike or kick may be forceful enough to knock the breath out of the person. Breathing will be difficult for a few seconds because of spasms of the chest muscles, but no specific therapy is needed since regular breathing will return when the spasms disappear. Applying ice to the bruised area will relieve swelling and pain.

Female participants can sustain breast injuries during sparring, which is not unusual, but it can be serious since the breast is made up of loose, fatty tissue and bleeding into the breast can be more extensive. Breast injuries should be treated by immediately applying ice, and a wide elastic wrap should be used to relieve swelling and control internal bleeding. It should be left on for 24 hours with ice packs applied for 20-minute periods over the elastic wrap three times a day. Training should then be delayed until swelling and tenderness in the injured breast have subsided. A firm well-supported brassiere should be used during future workouts.

COSTO CHONDRAL INJURIES

Costo chondral injuries can occur when a blow is received on the cartilage junctions of the rib (see illustration #18) which are located about 2″ on each side of the sternum. A forceful blow causes an injury to the ligamentous structure holding the rib to the cartilage. Pain is increased by deep breathing, coughing or sneezing. Carefully feeling the area with the fingertips will reveal a very tender region over the cartilage and rib junction. It will often be misdiagnosed as a rib fracture. Treatment of costo chondral injuries is similar to the treatment for rib fractures. The injured area should be iced for 20 minutes, three times a day for the first three days

THE TRUNK

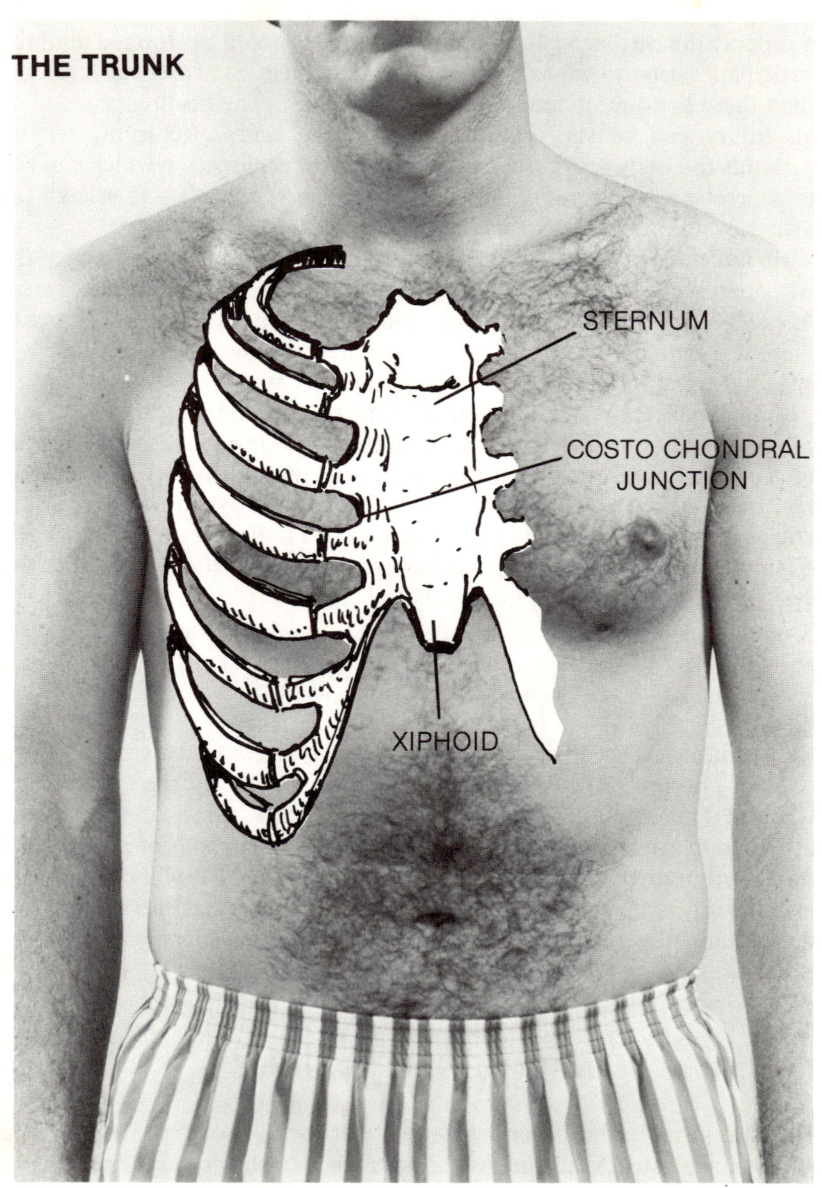

ILLUSTRATION # 18

to relieve pain, and then an elastic rib belt should be worn around the chest to support the cartilage-rib junction. Workouts should be stopped until the participant feels no more pain in the chest area. Sparring may resume when there is no more tenderness over the chest. The healing process for this injury can be very slow and painful at times. Returning to full workouts too early only results in an inflammed rib junction which can last for several weeks, or months. When this occurs, consult a physician for further evaluation and treatment.

Rib injuries can occur in both karate and judo-type activities. Again, the participant will have received a punch or kick or a knee to the chest area. This will be followed by severe pain and an inability to catch one's breath. There will be pain at the site of the fractured rib and the participant will only find relief by holding or bracing the chest wall with his hands.

Immediate treatment should be directed toward splinting the chest wall with a rib belt or an elastic wrapping. Instructors should advise students to refrain from further activity and seek medical help when they suspect a rib fracture. Healing will usually take six weeks, and when the participant returns to sparring, a chest pad should be worn until there is no tenderness over the rib injury site. Judo practitioners should not return to practice until all pain and tenderness have subsided.

CARDIAC INJURIES

Heart injuries, usually due to a blow to the chest, are rare, especially in a well-run gym setting or tournament. But it is still wise for the instructor to be aware that such injuries can occur. In most cases, there will usually be a loss of consciousness by the injured participant as a result of an irregular heart rhythm or from cardiac arrest. In either case, CPR will be necessary until the injured person is in the hands of trained medical personnel. It is wise to remember that powerful blows to the chest can cause heart injuries. (See Chapter One for CPR instructions.)

ABDOMINAL INJURIES

Most injuries to the abdominal wall are bruises. A solar plexus blow is a punch or kick struck just below the sternum into the *epigastric* portion of the abdomen (see illustration #20). This is known as a knockout area in boxing as well. A well-directed blow to the area causes a sudden drop in blood pressure and a slowing of the pulse. There is also an accompanying loss of breath due to abdominal wall muscle spasms. Treatment should be directed toward supporting the blood pressure.

Placing the injured person on his back and raising the legs about 18″ to 24″ above the floor is usually helpful, and if the abdominal wall is in spasm, the knees should be flexed toward the chest after the participant is on his back. This will relieve the spasm and pain and help restore more normal breathing. No other treatment is usually necessary.

A hard fall to the floor from a judo throw or a karate foot sweep may cause an internal abdominal injury. The major point to be made here is that any intra-abdominal injury is usually a surgical emergency. Because of this, the instructor must be alert and aware of this type of injury. Any student or participant who receives a forceful blow to the abdominal area with subsequent severe abdominal pain must see a doctor immediately. Persistent abdominal pain, abdominal tenderness, pallor, clamminess, a shocky appearance, nausea and weakness are all signs of a serious internal

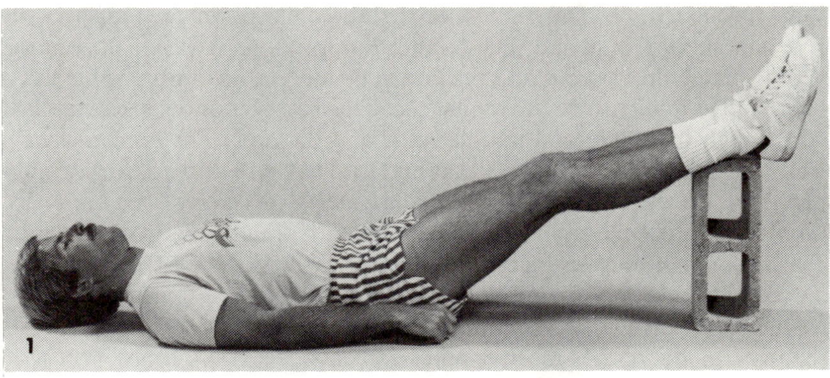

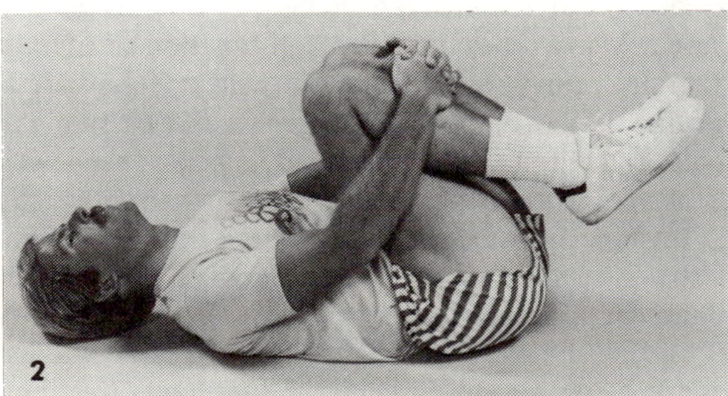

ILLUSTRATION # 19

If a person receives a blow to the abdomen, place them on their back (1) and raise their legs 18″ to 24″ above the floor. If the injury is to the groin (2) have them bring their knees toward the chest to relieve any spasms.

injury. If these symptoms do not disappear within a few seconds, the participant should be transferred immediately to a medical center by ambulance for surgical evaluation.

Injuries to the testicles are rare and should never occur in the martial arts when proper equipment and supervision are used. But when it happens, the person should be placed on his back, and he should gently flex his knees toward his chest to help relieve abdominal wall spasms. Once that is done, ice packs should be applied to the scrotum to reduce swelling and bleeding around the testicles. Persistent swelling and pain in the scrotal sac should be evaluated by a physician.

LOWER BACK INJURIES

The lumbar spine and its accompanying soft-tissue structures are prone to strains and sprains in martial arts activities. Fractures and disc injuries are relatively uncommon in karate, but they may be more frequent in judo-type activities. The motion of the lower back, which comprises the five lumbar vertebrae and their connection to the *sacrum* (see illustration #20) is mainly in forward and backward bending. The lumbar spine has a very limited ability to rotate on its axis. This rotary motion is accomplished through the upper and middle spine and the hips. The lumbar area is well supplied with a heavy muscular and ligament structure to carry the upper torso on the pelvis. The heavy muscular structures of the back also provide the internal organs of the abdomen from attacks from the rear. The abdominal muscles stabilize the lower back from the front and also aid the limiting motion of the back in back bending. Instructors and trainers must always keep in mind the development of the front as well as the back of the body's muscles and ligaments.

Strains in the lower back occur from overstretching or overtaxing the muscles in the lumbar area. Many times there is a combination of muscle (strain) and ligament (sprain) injury in this area. To help differentiate a strain injury from a sprain, the instructor and trainer should be familiar with these basic principles. When evaluating a strained muscle of the lower back, it is useful to feel the area where the martial arts participant points to as the site of the pain. Pushing into the affected injured muscle will increase the pain if it is a strain. A ligament injury will usually not be tender to the touch since the ligament structures lie deeper. Asking the student to bend to the right while resisting the motion to right with your hand will increase the pain in a strain but not in a sprain. This applies in all directions

ILLUSTRATION # 20

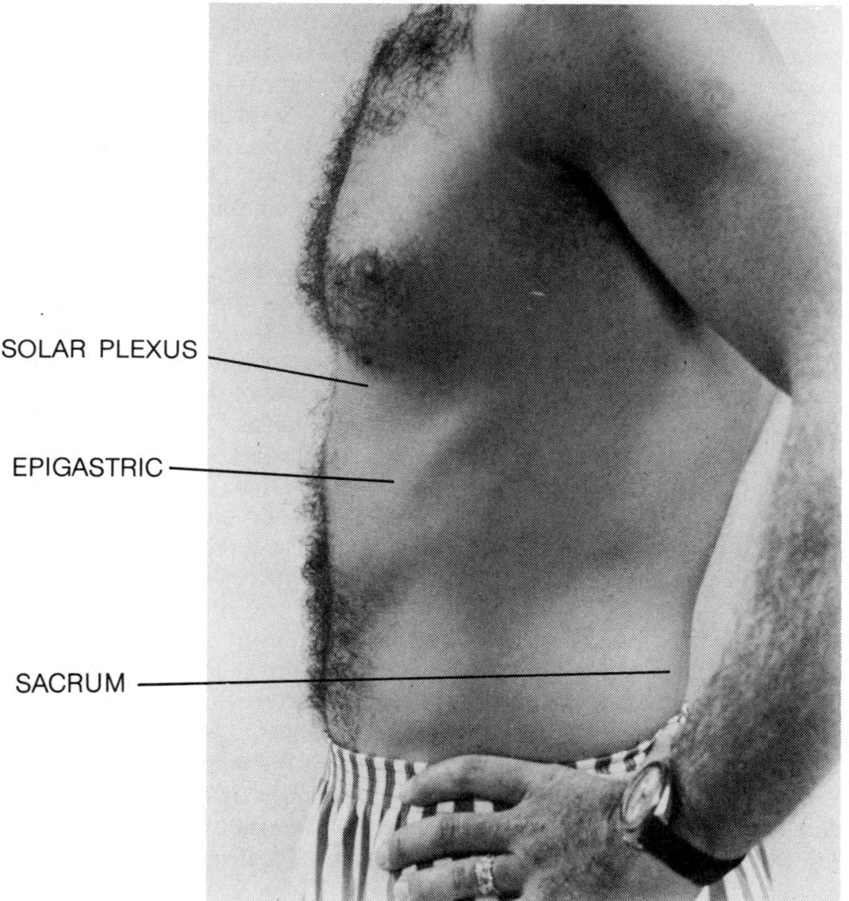

THE TRUNK (SIDE VIEW)

of the back except in a forward direction. Pain will also occur when the injured back muscle is overstretched. The range of motion of the spine, if done very slowly, will not be restricted in a pure strain-type injury of the spine in contrast to a sprain where any motion of the spine will increase the pain.

Now that you have a basic idea of how to evaluate a strain of the lower back, how do you treat it? Strains should be treated immediately with ice application to the tender area for the first 72 hours. Ice packs should be applied for 20 to 30 minutes, three times a day. Complete rest of the area is required until a full range of motion and freedom from pain in the back is restored. If it hurts, it is still injured and more time is required. The main causes of chronic injuries and complications are haste and hurry. There is no one contest or tournament important enough to cause a permanent injury. Never push yourself into a situation which will increase an already present injury. An old physician axiom is "the best healer is the tincture of time." Martial arts is a way of life, not a rush to victory. In other words, rest the injured back until motion of the back is painless. This is not to be confused with the stiffness of inactivity. As soon as the back is pain-free, begin stretching exercises in a slow, methodical manner. Do not jerk or force the muscles. Gentle, slow stretching will restore the normal range of motion of the back without reinjury. Once you have restored the full range of motion to the area, you may return to your normal training schedule.

In some martial arts groups, it is a common practice to use manipulation procedures in back injuries. If the pain is mild and there is no question of a fracture, this is probably not harmful. However, do not use this type of approach to acute back injuries unless you have information available (such as X-rays) to rule out the presence of a fracture or a possible disc injury.

Sprains of the back involve injuries to the ligament of the back. They are more serious and require more time to recover. Again, as outlined in Chapter One, a sprain can range from mild-to-severe with a complete tearing of the ligament away from its boney attachment. This type of injury occurs when the normal range of movement of the intervertebral joint is exceeded. Immediate pain will usually be experienced in this type of injury following a bending or twisting movement. Movement of the spine following this injury will be painful in all directions, and motion will be decreased in all directions.

The treatment of lumbar sprains involves resting the injured ligament. There is always a great deal of muscle spasm present in an acute ligament injury. This is a physiological protection mechanism to keep the ligament from being moved. In other words, nature is saying, "Stop moving this part until it is healed."

Immediate treatment of an acute sprain is discontinuation of activity followed by immediate ice application to the painful area, as with strains. Bed rest will usually be required because of the severity of pain. After 72 hours, heat will provide a relieving effect. Two aspirin taken four times a day will help decrease pain and any accompanying inflammation. A firm bed or bed boards placed under the mattress will be helpful in keeping the back aligned in a neutral position during the recovery phase. Severe pain will require muscle relaxants and strong analgesics from a physician. All back injuries which produce severe pain or decreased ability in motion should be evaluated by your physician. Because of the slow healing time of ligament injuries, there will be a delay in the return to normal training exercises.

It is important that the injured martial artist does not return to floor exercises or competition until he has regained the full range of motion and strength in his lower back, and not until he is pain-free. ∎

CHAPTER 6
LOWER EXTREMITY INJURIES

THIGH INJURIES

Thigh injuries in the martial arts usually involve the large muscular portion in the front of the leg (the *quadriceps*) or the back of the thigh (the *hamstrings*). A common injury to the quadriceps is a bruise, which usually occurs from kicks to the thigh. Bleeding and swelling should be controlled immediately by applying ice and then placing an elastic wrap on the thigh. Both should continue for up to 72 hours, with ice being applied for 20-minute periods, three times a day.

The time when a student can return to activity will depend on the severity of the bruise, which can be gauged by the ability to flex the knee fully without pain. If there is pain in the thigh muscles when the knee is bent, it is advised to delay returning to practice. When full flexion is possible without pain, it is safe to begin practice. It is a poor practice to rub or massage a bruise on the thigh during the early period of the injury (i.e., the first seven to ten days). This is especially true with a deep bruise which includes bleeding.

Massage during this healing period has been shown to produce a complication called *myositis ossificans,* which is believed to occur because of stimulation of the *periosteum* (the cellular lining of the bone). When this occurs, a boney mass develops in the injured area of the muscle. Prematurely returning to practice or improperly massaging this injury results in an increased growth of the bone mass. Any firm, hard mass felt in a deep bruise in a muscle injury should be evaluated by a physician. X-rays will reveal a fairly typical picture of calcium deposits in the muscle tissue. Treatment requires rest to the injured part and protection from further injury. The calcium deposits usually disappear from the muscle tissue after a time: therefore, surgery for this condition is seldom necessary.

In the martial arts, strains can occur in the groin muscles or hamstrings of the thigh when there was not a sufficient warm-up period. It is especially important that stretching and flexibility calisthenics precede all regular classwork and sparring.

Strains of the groin or the hamstring muscle group are easily recognized. There will usually be immediate pain or tightness felt at the site of the injury. Pain and tightness will increase as the practitioner continues to use the injured part. Feeling around the injured area will help find any tenderness in the strained muscle, and the athlete will feel pain in the back of the thigh while doing certain movements such as front kicks; groin injuries will cause discomfort with such motions as side kicks.

BONES AND MUSCLES OF THE LEG

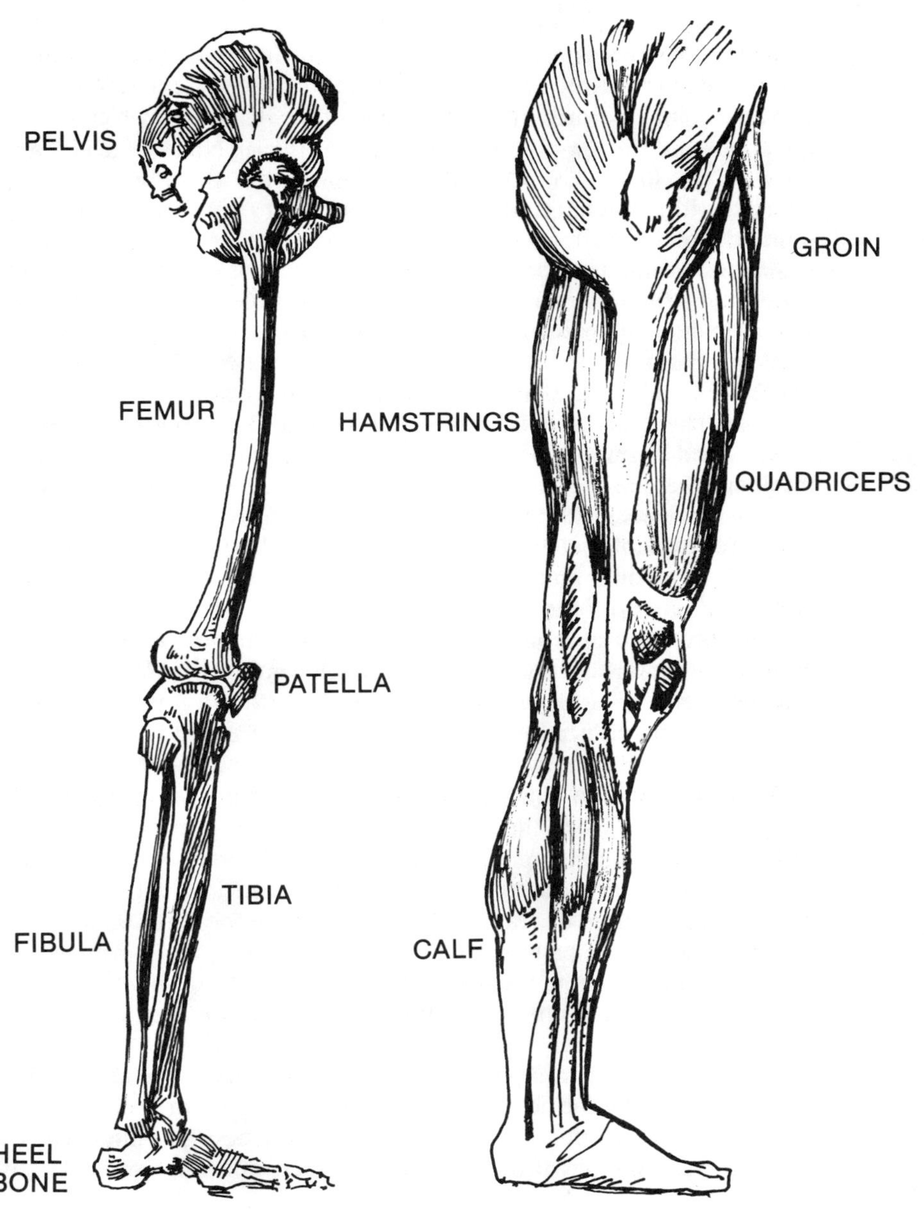

ILLUSTRATION # 21

KNEE INJURIES

The knee joint is the largest joint in the body and the most susceptible to injury. The knee is protected from injury by its basic boney configuration forming the joint, by its ligaments and by the surrounding muscles. The knee joint is formed by the lower end of the thigh bone which is called the *femur* and the upper end of the larger of the leg bones which is called the *tibia* (see illustration #21). The ends of each of these bones are constructed with smooth, connecting surfaces, and they form a hinge-type joint which is held together by strong ligaments as well as muscle attachments around the knee. The kneecap is a part of the knee joint, and it consists of a *sesamoid* bone arising in the tendon of the quadriceps muscle of the thigh. The kneecap provides a protective boney covering over the front of the knee joint. Within the joint lie two *fibrocartilagenous semilunar* (semi-moon shaped) cartilages, which are attached to the top of the tibia. These cartilages help to spread the joint fluid over the connecting surfaces and to smooth out any irregularities of the connecting surface of the joint. Despite the fact the cartilages are attached to the tibia, functionally they move with the femur, which is the reason they are injured so often. For example, when the knee is straightened, the cartilages glide forward with the femur on the tibia, and when the knee is bent, the cartilages glide backward with the femur on the tibia.

Basically, injuries around the knee fall into four general categories: 1) bruises; 2) strains involving muscle attachments; 3) sprains involving ligaments; and 4) cartilage injuries. There is a fifth category which would be fractures and dislocations, but these occur so infrequently in the martial arts that they have not even been included in this handbook.

The most common injury is a bruise occurring from a low kick or from using the knee to block the kick. Usually the boney heel or the forefoot strike the knee, causing minor bleeding in the soft tissue around the knee, leaving a tender, bruised area. These are best treated by immediately applying ice to the injured area, which should be done for 15 to 20 minutes. It will markedly reduce pain, stiffness and swelling later, and it will help the practitioner maintain his training schedule without lost time. Ice application should then continue two or three times a day for the first 72 hours after the injury occurs.

Another common injury is a hyperextension injury to the knee. This is usually suffered by the novice martial arts practitioner, or it occurs in the advanced student during sparring or competitive action. The injury can occur during a front kick if the knee joint is forced to straighten beyond its

THE KNEE

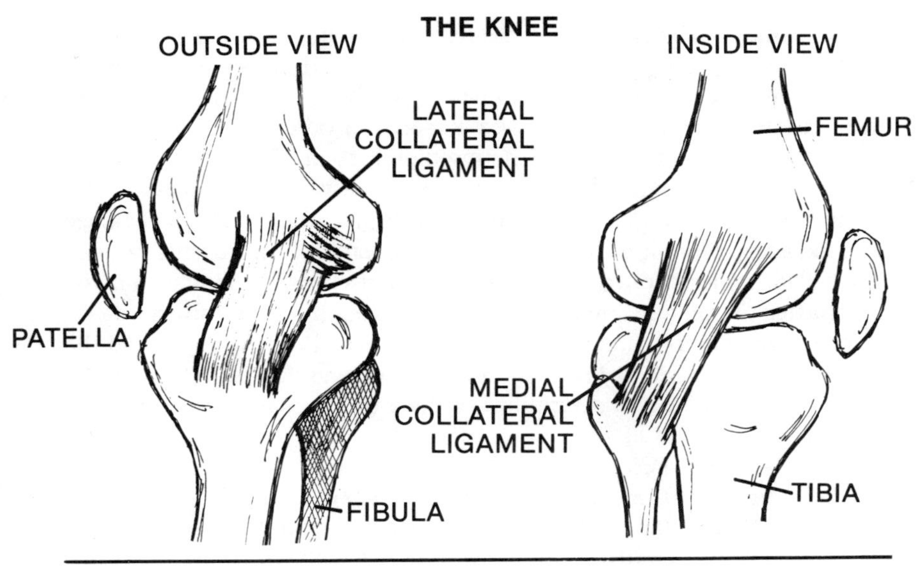

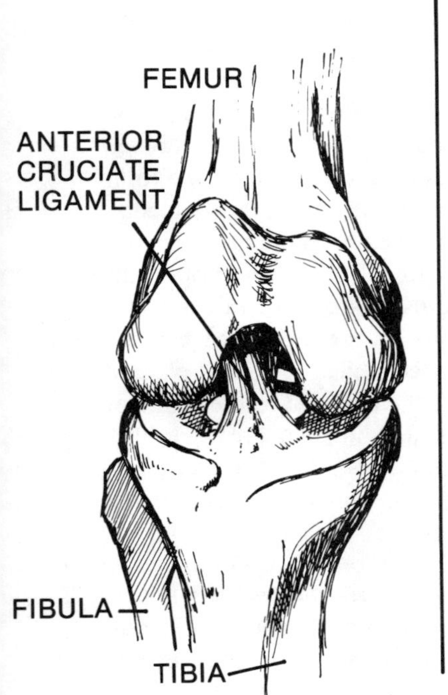

FRONT VIEW OF KNEE JOINT

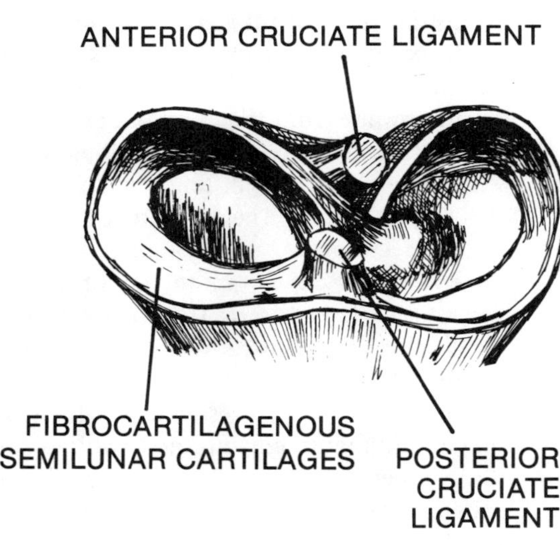

TOP VIEW OF KNEE JOINT

ILLUSTRATION # 22

normal range. When this occurs, the hamstring tendons at the back of the knee are usually overstretched, and there is usually immediate pain in the back of the knee. Treatment again involves applying ice to the most tender area and then wrapping an elastic bandage around the knee. Gently stretching the hamstring and restricting high kick motions for a few days after returning to training will help complete the recovery process.

Another injury seen less commonly is an injury to the front of the knee in the kneecap tendon or in the thigh muscle tendon. This occurs by sudden violent contraction of the large thigh muscles after landing on the floor, after jumping techniques or after breaking a fall. Treatment again includes applying ice and an elastic wrap, and rest. Any injury around the tendons that has not subsided within a five-to-seven day period should be checked by a physican to determine if a more serious tear of the tendon is present.

Probably the most common injury to the knee is an injury to the medial (inside) collateral ligaments (see illustration #22). This is a much more serious debilitating injury than those previously mentioned because it involves the actual stability of the knee joint. Most often in tae kwon do, there is usually only a partial or incomplete tearing of the inside collateral ligament. Occasionally, however, a more complete tear occurs causing immediate disability with an unstable knee joint. Many of the minor sprains of the inside collateral ligament again occur in the less experienced student while executing the side kick, which requires raising the knee prior to executing the side thrust. If the knee is not raised to a proper height, the leg snaps upward from the knee and exerts pressure to the inside of the joint and ligaments. This causes stretching and tearing of the inside ligaments. There must be a straight-line thrust force from the hip to the heel to avoid this type of injury. The elevation of the knee, therefore, is very important in the execution of the sidekick and in avoiding this type of injury.

The other most common way to injure this ligament occurs when the practitioner is kicked on the outside of the knee while the foot is planted on the floor (see illustration #23). The force is then exerted to the inside of the knee, thereby stretching the inside collateral ligaments. Treatment for the minor sprain involves icing, elastic wraps and rest. A moderate sprain may require immobilizing the knee in a splint for four-to-six weeks while the ligaments heal. And a complete tear requires surgical repair, and it should be repaired within a few days to get a good-functioning, stable knee. If the injury is repaired after a week or more, the result is not as satisfactory. For this reason, early diagnosis is most important. In any questionable, serious knee injury, it is always advisable to seek expert

ILLUSTRATION # 23

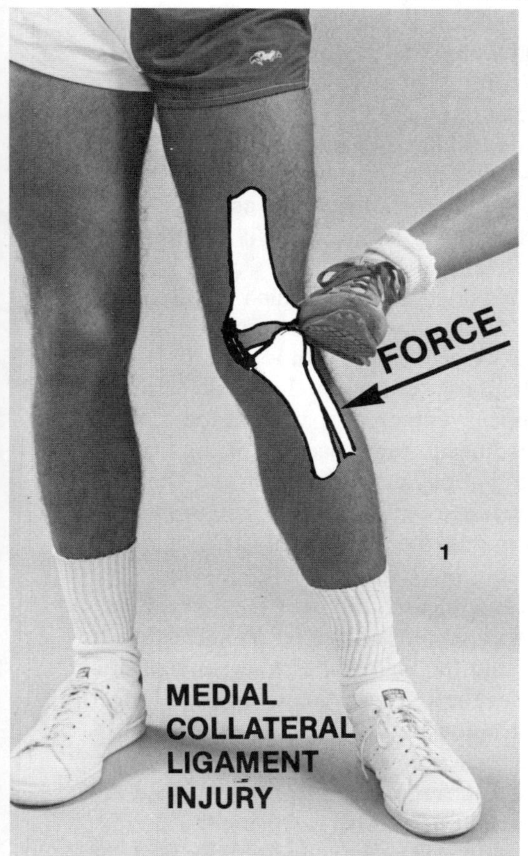

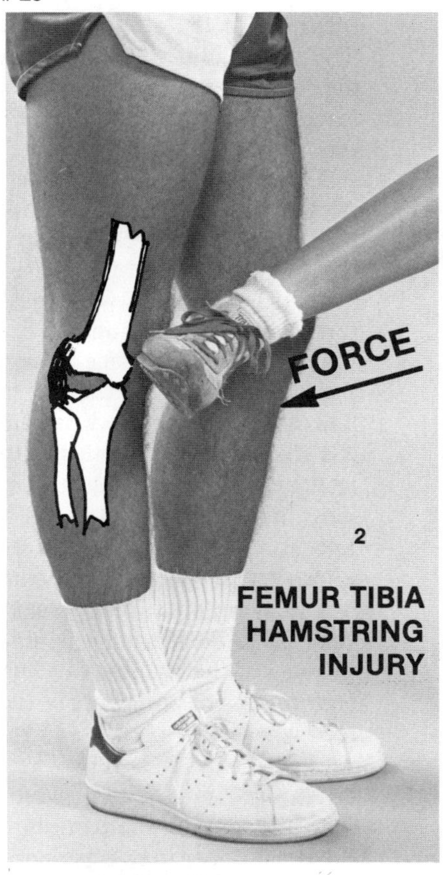

A common way to injure the ligaments of the knee is to receive a kick to that area. If the kick is from the outside (1), the medial (inside) ligaments are likely to be torn; and if the kick is from the front (2) the anterior ligaments in the back of the knee are likely to be torn. Treatment for a minor sprain (tear) will involve applying ice to the area, wrapping it and resting it. A moderate sprain will require immobilizing the knee in a splint for up to six weeks. A major sprain (a complete tear) will require surgical repair.

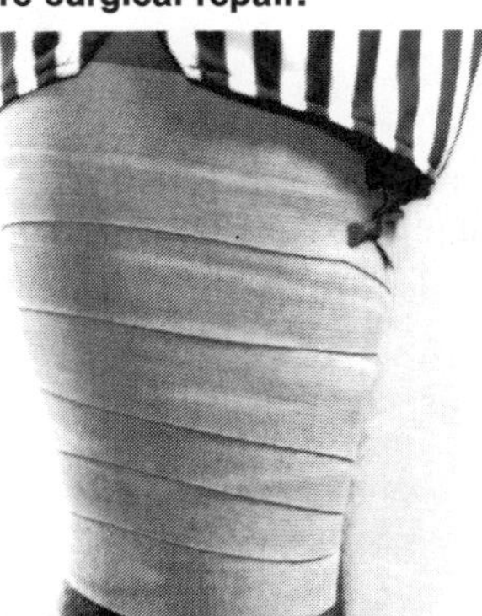

If the thigh receives a kick or blow, bleeding and swelling may be controlled by applying ice to the injury and then by (1) placing an elastic wrap around the thigh, which should be worn for up to three days after the injury occurs.

medical evaluation at once.

Injury to the outside collateral ligament is less common in karate activities. The injury is usually caused by a kick to the inside of the knee with the foot planted on the floor, or as a result of a sweep kick. This exerts a force to the outside collateral ligaments of the knee joint. Treatment is similar to what is done for the inside collateral ligament tear.

The *anterior cruciate* ligament, which lies within the knee joint can also be injured in a variety of ways. In martial arts activity, it is usually injured as a result of a direct blow to the front of the knee. This is a commonly overlooked ligament injury (see illustration #22).

Cartilage injuries in the knee occur due to activities which require rapid turning or twisting motions, or by a direct blow to the outside of the knee joint. A medial cartilage injury occurs when, as the foot is fixed firmly on the floor with the knees bent, the thigh rotates toward the inside or center line of the body, and when that happens with great speed and force, there is a vigorous stress applied to the medial cartilage. Because of the firm attachment of the medial cartilage to that collateral ligament and the tibia itself, a rupture or splitting of the cartilage can occur if the rotation of the knee joint continues beyond its normal limits. The lateral cartilage of the knee, due to its greater mobility within the joint, is seldom injured.

The symptoms which result from a medial cartilage tear are all too familiar to the martial arts practitioner who has suffered from this injury because of the extreme swelling around the knee joint. Another sign of a torn cartilage is a locking sensation of the knee. At times, the practitioner may experience locking and sudden unlocking of the knee as the joint is rotated. This is caused by a torn portion of the cartilage being trapped between the joint formed by the tibia and femur. Following a cartilage injury, the swelling and pain subside within a few weeks. During this period, the practitioner may experience a giving way or buckling sensation of the knee. He may also notice recurrent swelling and stiffness of the knee after exercise. Treatment of a torn cartilage is usually surgery by an orthopedic specialist to remove the cartilage. Early conservative treatment consists of elastic wraps, ice application and rest of the knee joint until swelling and pain disappear.

ANKLE INJURIES

The ankle joint is basically a hinge joint constructed to allow up and down motions and a certain degree of rotation. There are three groups of

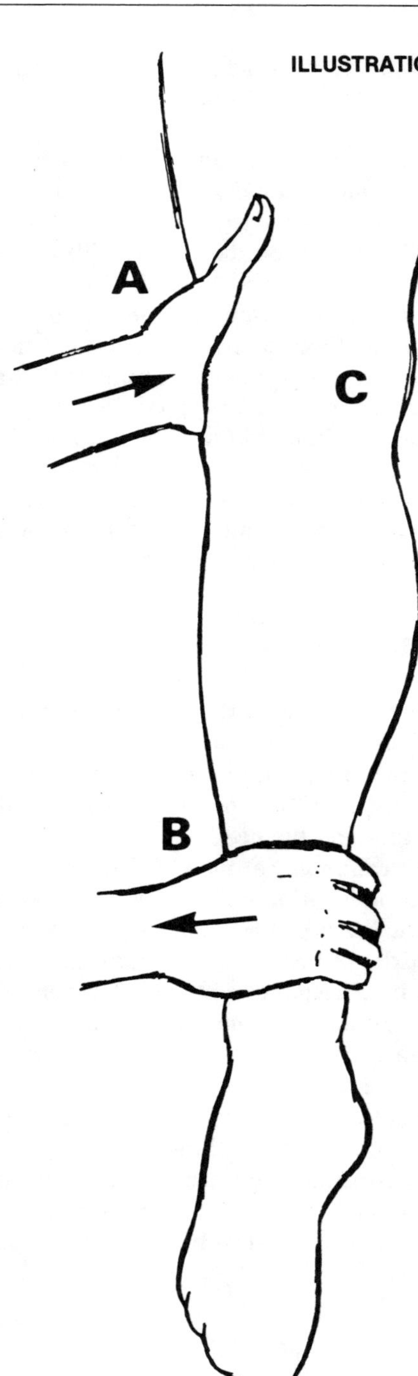

Hand A applies pressure to the outside of the knee joint while hand B grasps the ankle and force is applied outward. When a mild tear is present, pain is experienced at C. If there is an extensive tear of the medial ligament, there will be noted a gapping or opening sensation of the joint at C. To test the lateral ligament the pressure is applied to the inside of the knee joint with hand A and inward force is applied with hand B.

ligaments that support the ankle joint: A large ligamentous band on the outside, a ligament on the inside, and a ligament on the back side of the ankle (see illustration #26).

The most common injury to the ankle is a sprain of the outside ligament, which is its weakest part. To demonstrate that weakness, turn your foot inward so it rests on the outside edge of the foot. Now push down on the foot and notice how unstable the ankle is on the outside with the foot in this position.

Ankle sprains can vary from a minimal first-degree injury to a severe third-degree tear. It is not the purpose of this handbook to give a detailed treatment of ankle injuries since it is a complex subject, but simple first-aid treatment of any ankle injury requires immediately applying ice to reduce swelling and bleeding, and then this should be followed by a compressive wrap with an elastic bandage. The ankle should then be elevated and it is a good idea to avoid putting too much weight on the injured joint until it can be evaluated by a physician. Under no circumstances should heat be applied to a joint injury during the first 72 hours. After that, it is actually a good idea.

FOOT INJURIES

The foot is one of the most important parts of the body in karate-type activities, since it serves as an offensive weapon as well as a defensive force. Because of the unique use of the foot in martial arts, it is more prone to injury than in other contact sports, and the type of injury is also different since it involves mostly the toes and the heel.

In karate, foot bruises occur most commonly around the toes, the heads of the metatarsals, or the heel (see illustration #27). When the toes are flexed upward as in a front kick, the heads of the metatarsals become the striking surface much like the knuckles of the fist. The metatarsals can be injured when striking a hard boney prominence or a hard surface while doing breaking techniques. The more serious, commonly-injured areas are the first (large toe) and second metatarsal heads, since they are larger and longer and make first contact with the target.

Treatment of bruises to the metatarsal heads consists of applying ice to them, wrapping them with elastic compressions, and then elevating them. Putting any weight on the injured part should be restricted until pain and swelling subside which is usually within 72 hours. A felt or foam pad can be strapped on the foot over the injured metatarsal heads to relieve pain during walking.

ILLUSTRATION # 26

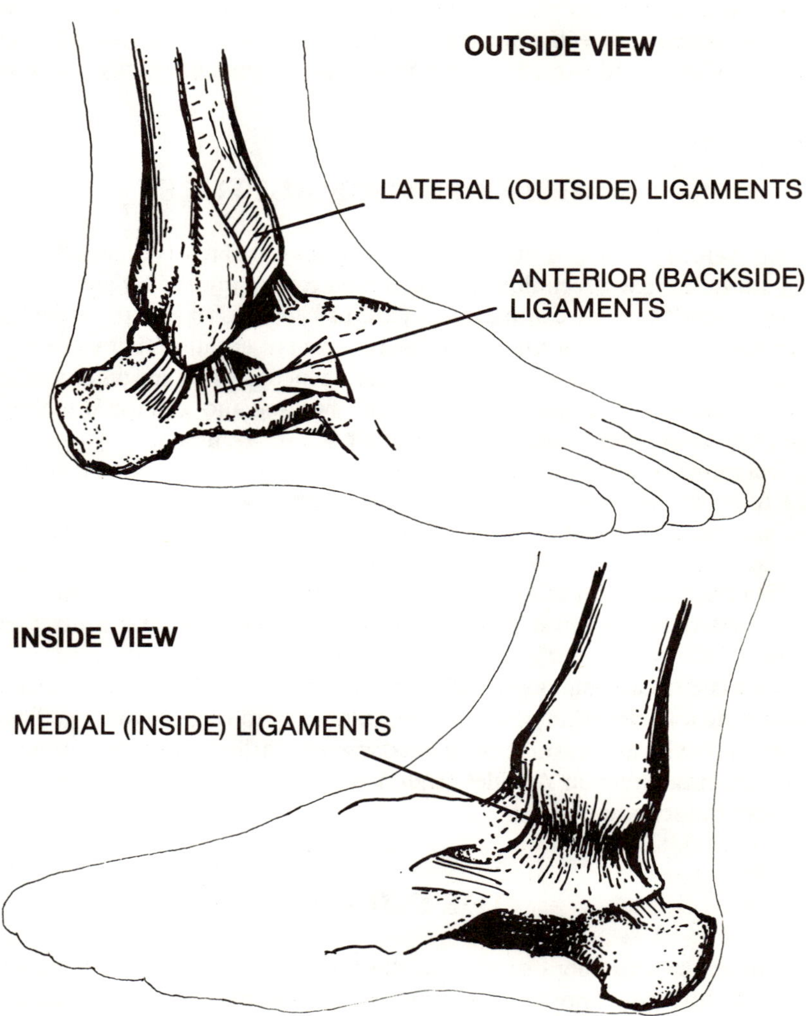

THE ANKLE

Heel bruises occur as a result of kicks which use the heel as a striking part (e.g., reverse roundhouse or back kicks). Treatment again consists of immediate ice application, compression and rest of the injured part. If pain and swelling persist in the metatarsal heads or heel area after five days, it is advised that the athlete consult his physician for possible X-ray examinations.

ACHILLES TENDON RUPTURE

An Achilles tendon rupture can occur in the martial arts especially during karate jumping techniques. The tendon can be injured by any sudden stress to the posterior compartment (calf or heel tendon group) of the leg.

The injury usually produces sudden pain and a sensation that something "popped" in the back of the heel tendon (which is often misdiagnosed as an ankle injury) and then there is usually swelling and a bluish discoloration appearing around the heel and ankle within 12 hours.

Diagnosis of a ruptured Achilles tendon can be made easier by making the following observations: 1) The injured person will not be able to stand on his toes; 2) When the calf muscle is gripped by the examiner's hand and squeezed, the foot will not flex downward, as it would normally; and 3) When the foot is dorsiflexed upward there is a depression of the heel tendon behind the ankle instead of the normal firm sensation of the intact tendon.

First-aid treatment consists of ice application to the injured area, elastic wrapping and elevation of the injured extremity to reduce swelling. These measures will aid a surgeon in making an earlier accurate diagnosis, because ultimately an Achilles tendon rupture requires surgical repair to restore the tendon.

TOE INJURIES

Toe injuries usually occur when the foot is blocked by an opponent's hand or forearm. Another way the toe may be injured is through improper positioning upon impact while executing a kick. Insufficient upward positioning of the toes causes excessive force to be applied to the joints of the toes. In a proper front kick, the metatarsal heads serve as the point of impact. The toes may also be injured when toes are forced into an over-flexed position. This results from improper execution of the kick with force being

ILLUSTRATION # 27

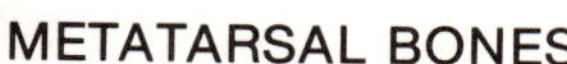

BONES OF THE FOOT

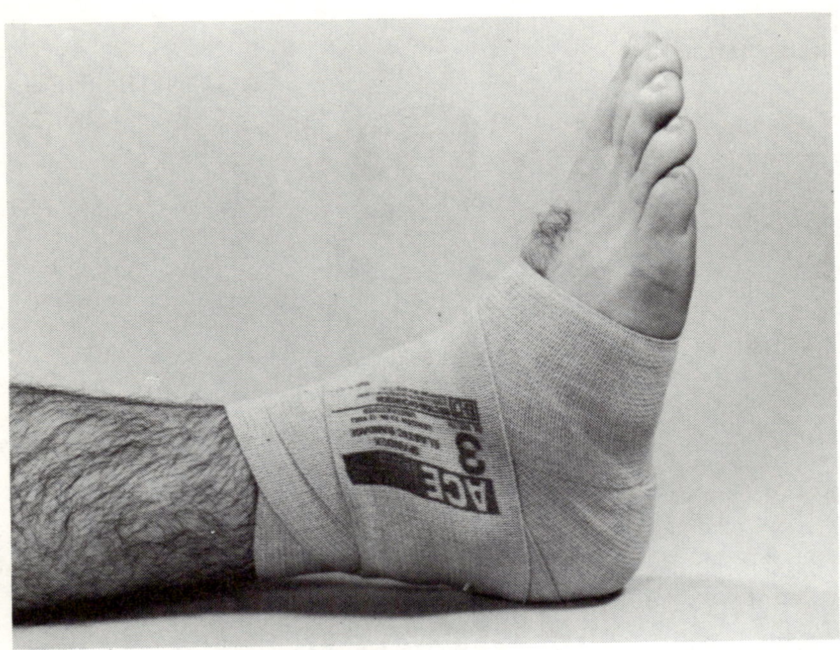

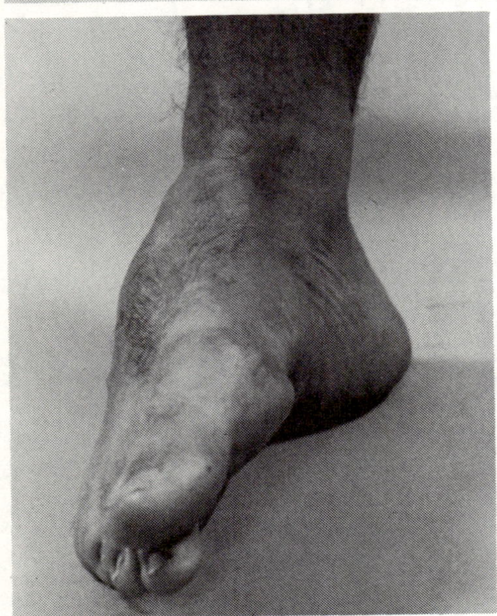

ILLUSTRATION # 28

WRAPPED ANKLE

If the ankle is injured, ice should be immediately applied to reduce swelling and bleeding, then the ankle should be wrapped with an elastic bandage, and it should be elevated.

ILLUSTRATION # 29

TESTING THE ANKLE

The outside ligament of the ankle is the weakest part of the foot. To demonstrate that weakness, turn your ankle inward so that it rests on the outside edge of the foot. Now push down with all your weight on that foot and notice how unstable it is.

applied to the tips of already flexed toes. This forces the toes into a hyperflexed position and results in a sprain, fracture, or dislocation of a toe or toes.

Toe injuries can best be avoided by using proper kicking techniques. Instructors should pay very particular attention to toe and foot positions when teaching kicking techniques. Sparring and breaking techniques should not be allowed until the instructor is absolutely sure the student is using the proper foot and toe position. This will reduce most of the common toe injuries encountered in karate-type activities.

When the metatarsal phalangeal joint is involved, a more extensive strapping is required to limit motion of the injured joint. First the injured toe is taped to the adjacent toe. The taping is then extended from the toes to the forefoot. Very little weight should be placed on the toes until the pain has subsided. A tennis shoe with the toe area cut out also offers some relief to this type of injury. The taping should be replaced daily and continued for at least a week or more to ensure proper healing of the injured joints. Persistent pain and swelling in the joints of the toes should be evaluated by a physician to rule out a fracture or tendon injury. ■

CHAPTER 7
REHABILITATION EXERCISES

It has been shown through studies that resting a soft-tissue injury only increases the probability that it will recur at the same site when activity resumes. Because of this, it is now recommended that the injured area be stretched up to the point of pain three times a day for about two minutes each time. This daily stretching causes stretching of scar-forming *collagen* fibers. When this is not done, the collagen tissue hardens into a glue-like consistency which renders the injured area into a rigid, inelastic state. This, in turn, makes the soft tissue more vulnerable to re-injury. It is estimated by Dr. William Stanish of the Royal College of Physicians and Surgeons that about 60 percent of activity-related injuries affect muscles, tendons and ligaments in people engaged in recreational sports who do not perform adequate warm-up and stretching exercises. Dr. Stanish advises an immediate stretching program be instituted following soft-tissue injuries. He also states any kind of stretching that involves the injury site promotes healing and flexibility.

NECK INJURIES

Neck exercises should be instituted soon (24 hours) after injury to help restore motion and relieve stiffness. These exercises and stretching motions are not recommended for severe neck injuries where there is a question of a nerve injury or vertebral fracture, which must be treated by a physician. It is to be understood, then, that these exercises are to be used only for soft-tissue injuries and minor sprains and strains.

HEAD ROTATION EXERCISE

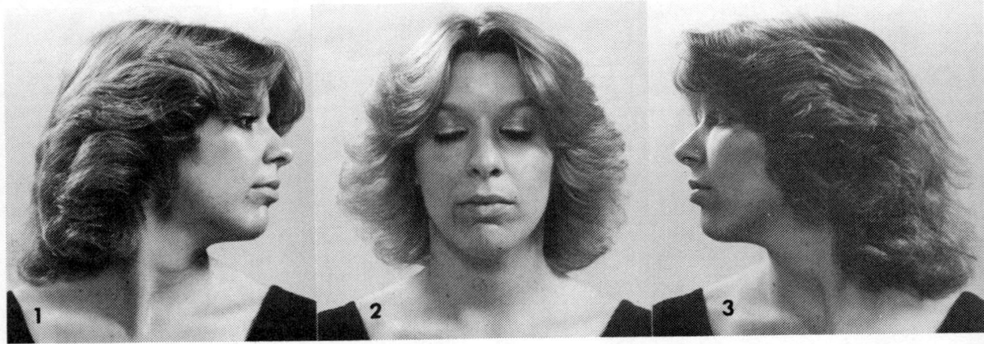

Slowly turn your head (1) as far as possible to the right. Then (2) return to the center position. Next (3) turn your head as far as possible to the left. Hold each of these positions for a ten-count.

HEAD FLEXION AND EXTENSION EXERCISE

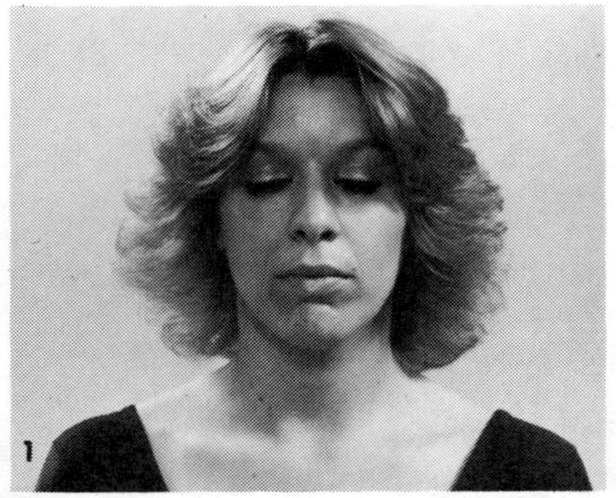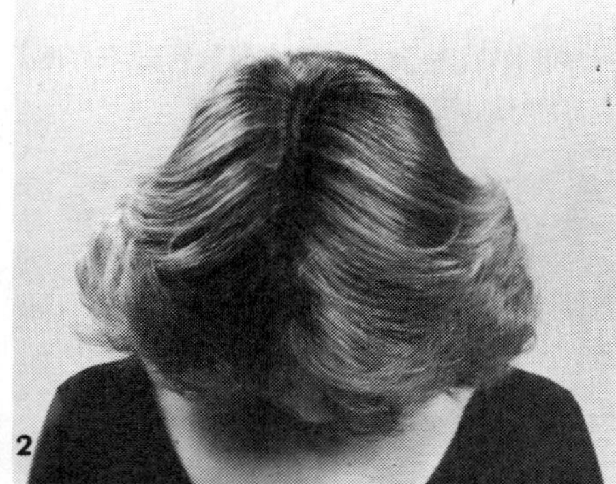

Stand or sit erect (1). Then (2) try to touch your chin to your chest. Do this slowly. If pain is experienced, your head should be brought back only to the point of pain until the motion becomes easier and without pain.

HEAD SIDE TILT EXERCISE

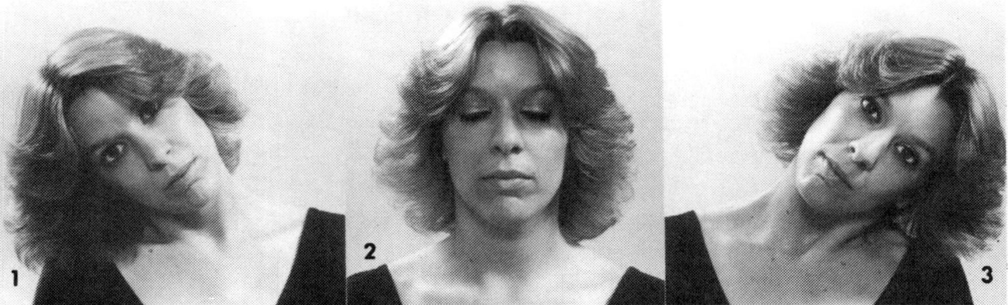

Try to touch your right ear (1) to your right shoulder. Return to the center position (2) and relax. Then (3) try to touch your left ear to your left shoulder. Hold each movement for a ten-count.

These three basic exercises are to be done until all motions are pain-free before progressing to more strenuous exercises. It is recommended that each exercise be performed ten times. When pain is lessened, then each exercise movement should be performed through the entire range of motion and continue to contract the neck muscles at the completion of the movement for an additional five seconds. For example, in the head rotation exercise, rotate the head slowly to the right as far as the head will turn and then contract the neck muscle for five seconds. Next, rotate the head slowly to the left and then repeat five seconds of contraction at the end of the motion. These exercises can be performed while standing under· a hot shower to increase relaxation and promote flexibility.

PENDULUM WEIGHT EXERCISE

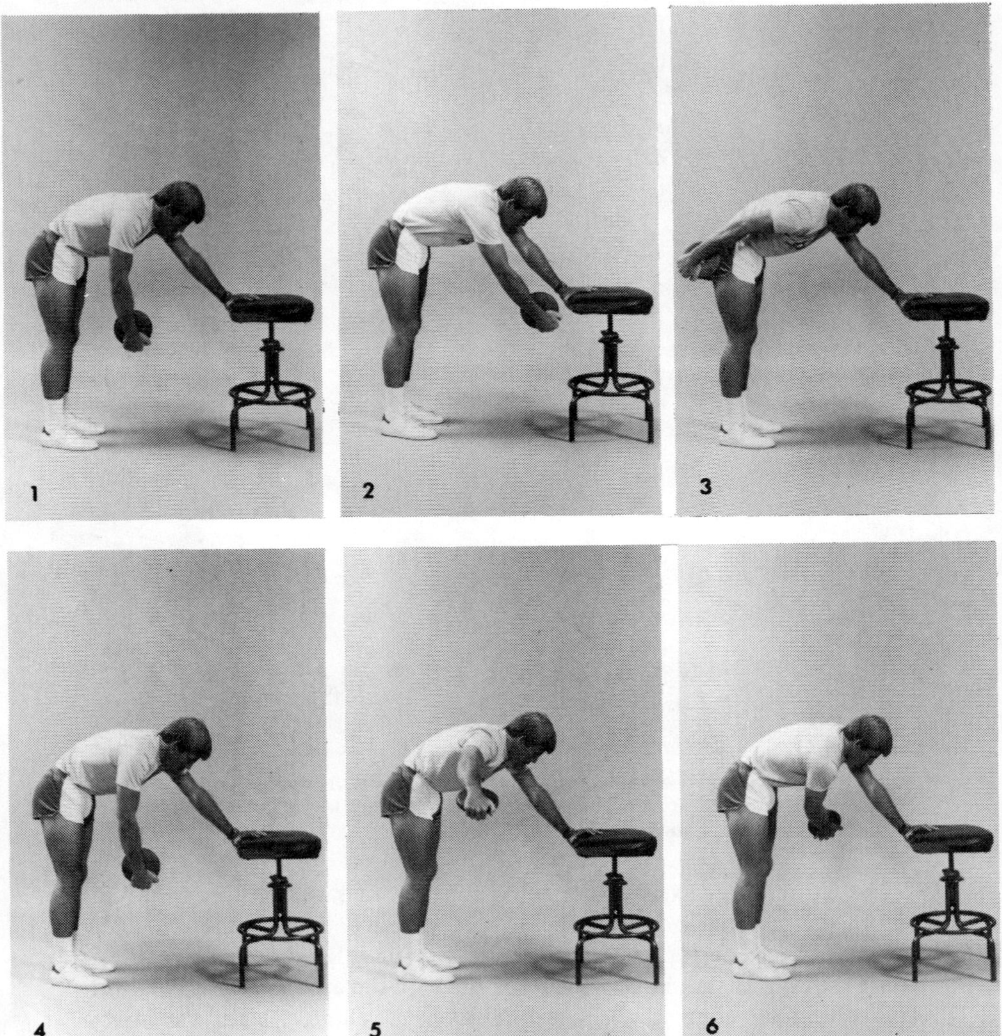

Lean forward and hold onto a table or stool (1) with the hand of the unaffected shoulder. Hold a one- or two-pound weight in the hand of the affected side. Relax the shoulders and let your arm hang loosely. Then swing the arm forward (2) and backward (3) with the elbow straight. Next, (4) swing your arm to the right (5) and then to the left (6). Do this exercise for about three minutes, two or three times a day. Generally, 25 swings in each direction will be adequate.

CODMAN WEIGHT EXERCISE

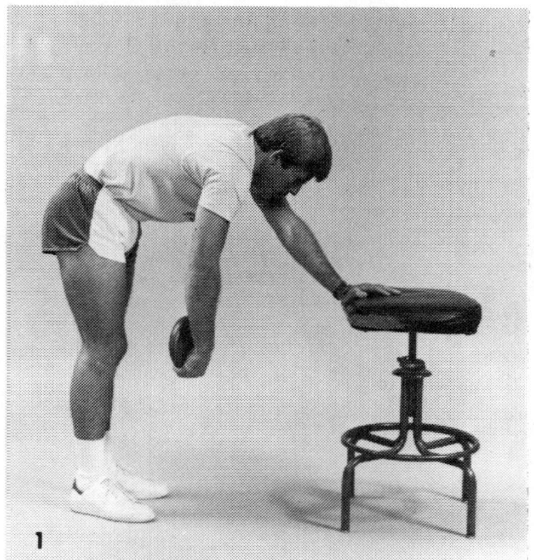 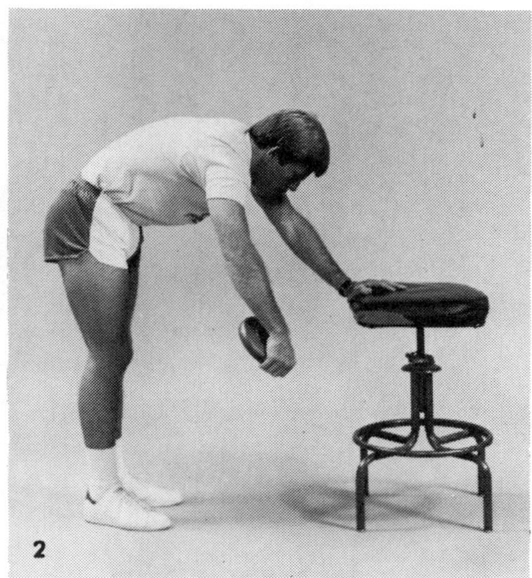

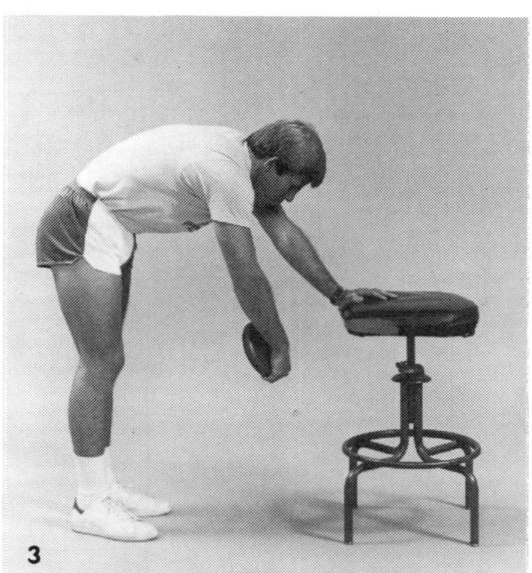 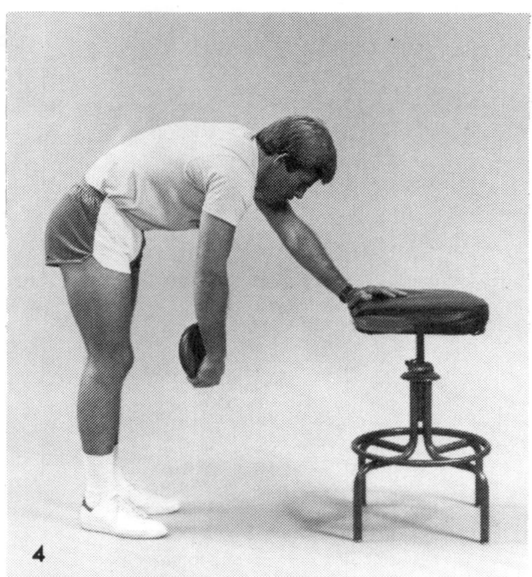

The Codman exercise is performed like the pendulum with the upper trunk bent forward (1) and the affected arm hanging down with the elbow straight.The arm is then moved (2-4) in a circular motion clockwise for 10-20 circles and then counterclockwise. As pain subsides in the shoulder, the circles should become wider in circumference.

LATERAL RAISES OVER THE HEAD

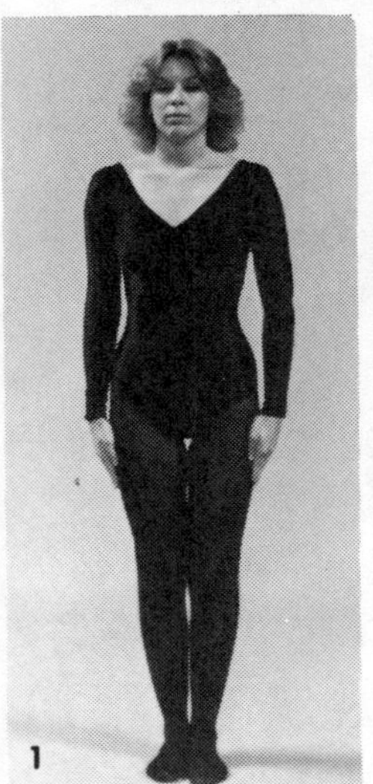 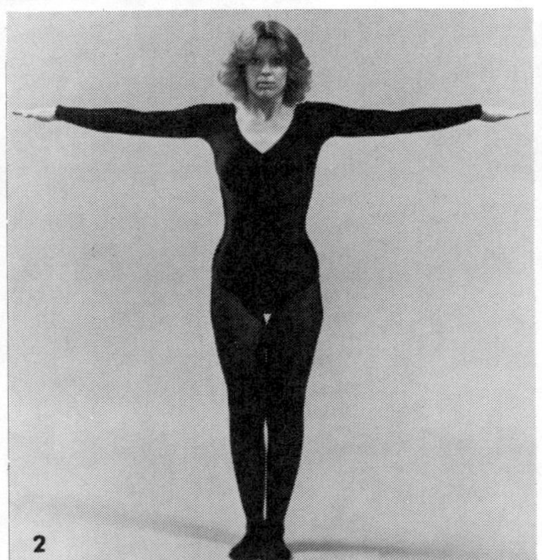 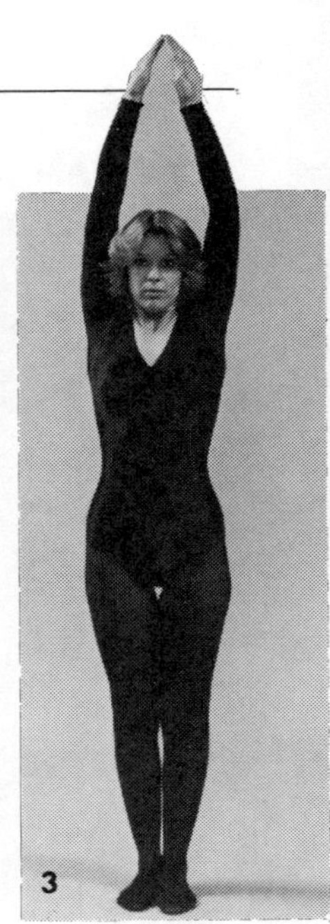

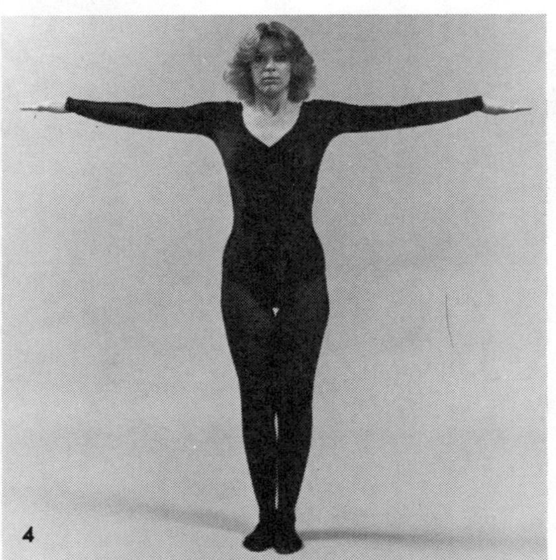 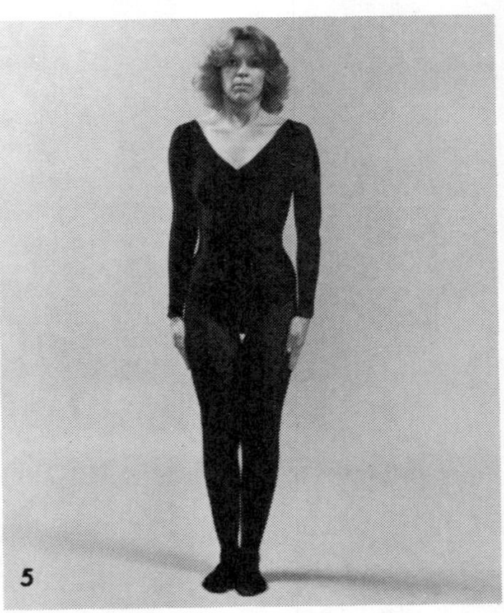

Stand (1) erect with your arms at your sides. Raise your arms (2) straight out to the sides. Then (3) bring your hands together over your head with your palms facing out. Lower your arms (4&5) to the sides again. Do this ten times. Then repeat the exercises with your palms turned in toward each other. Attempt to touch your palms at the top of your head.

FORWARD SWING EXERCISE

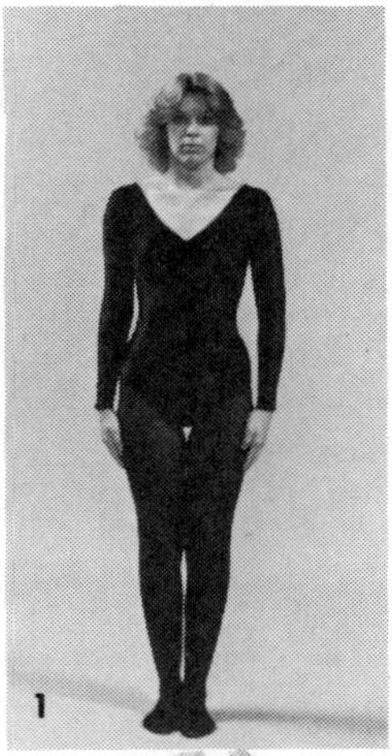
1

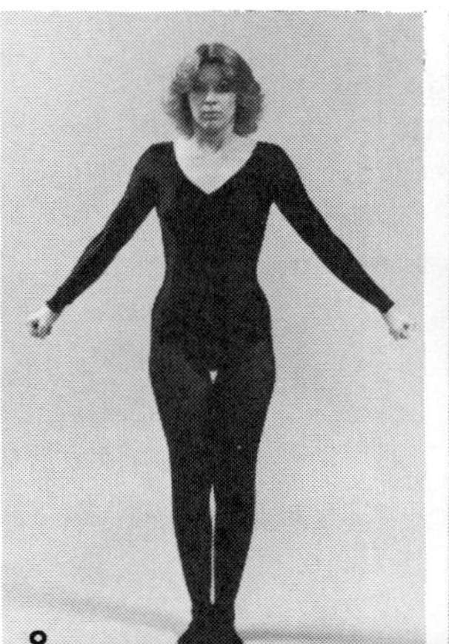

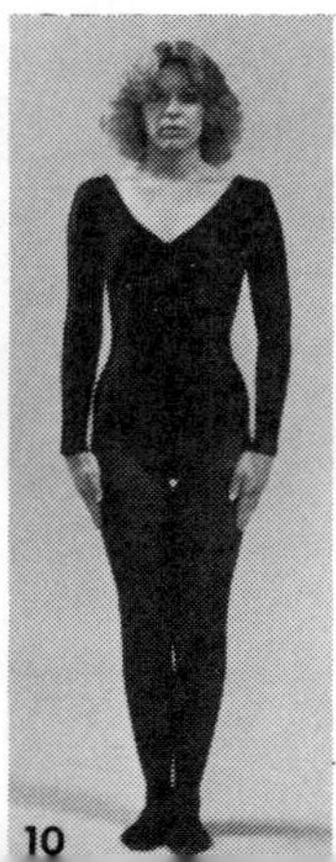

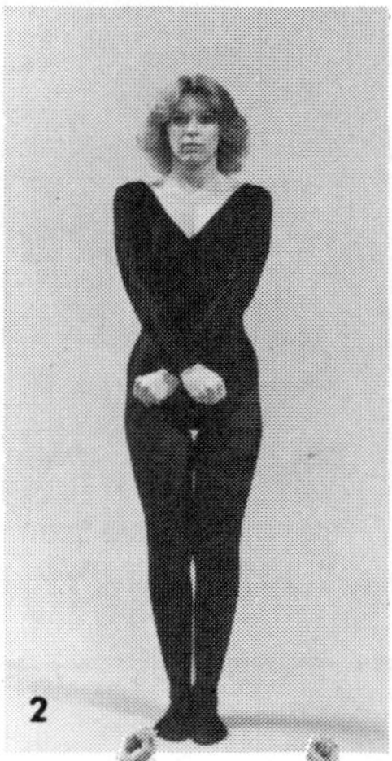
2

3

4

5

6

7

8

9

10

Standing erect (1) cross your wrists (2) in front of your body. Move your arms upward (3-5) keeping your elbows straight. Stretch your arms backward (6) above your head and uncross your wrists (7) as your arms move upward and outward. Then (8-10) lower your arms and return to the starting position. Do this movement ten times a day.

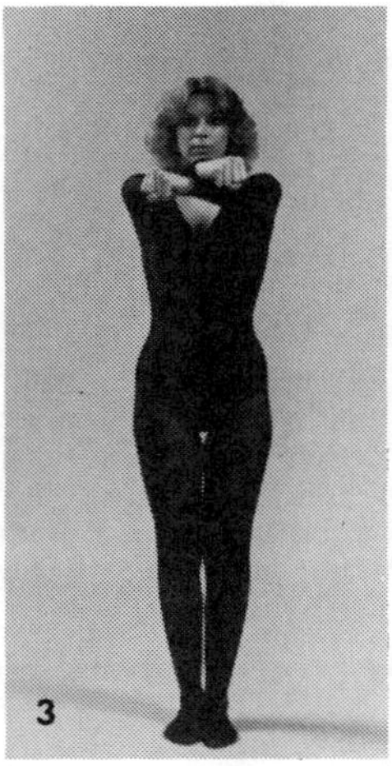

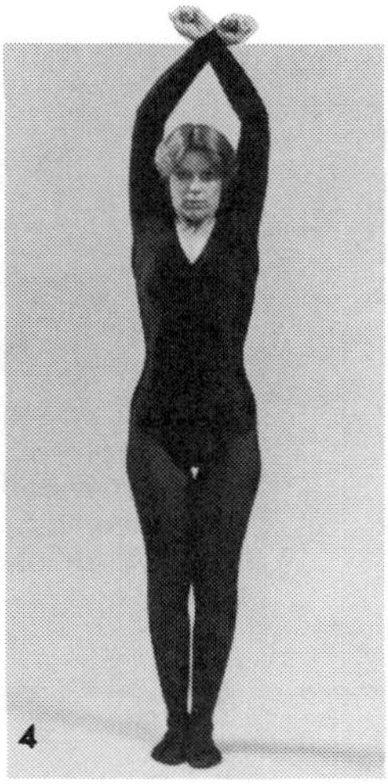

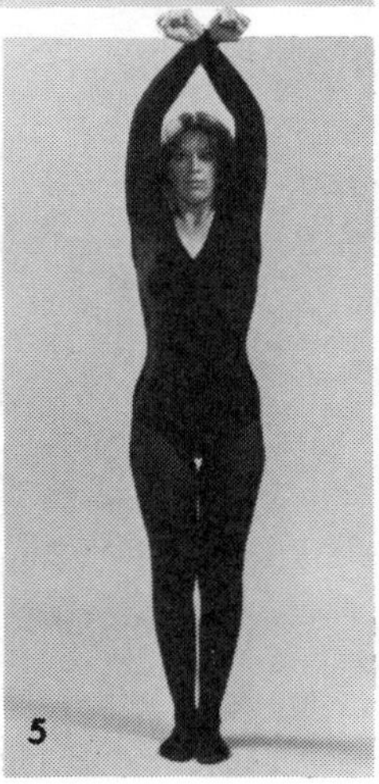

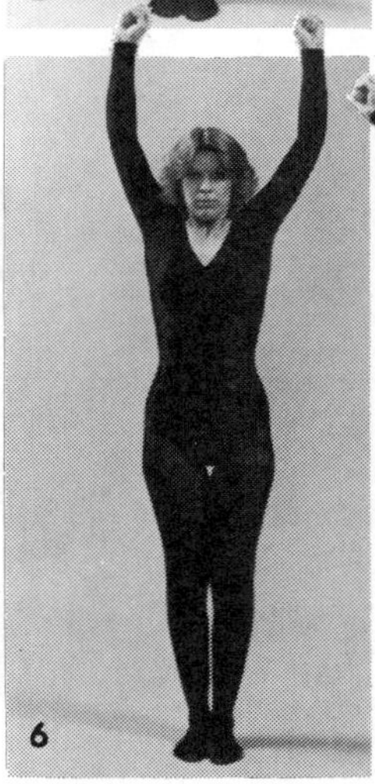

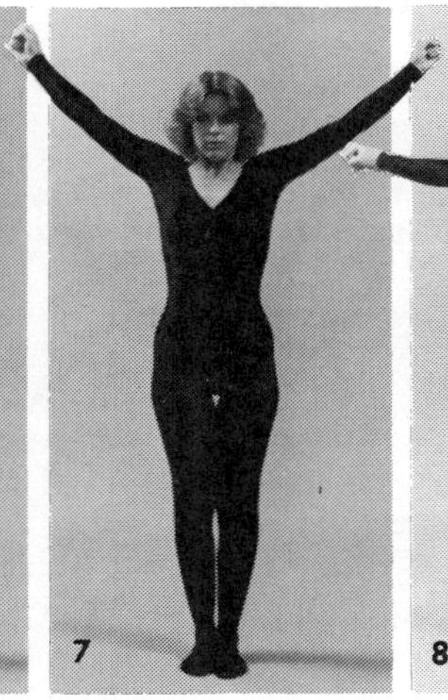

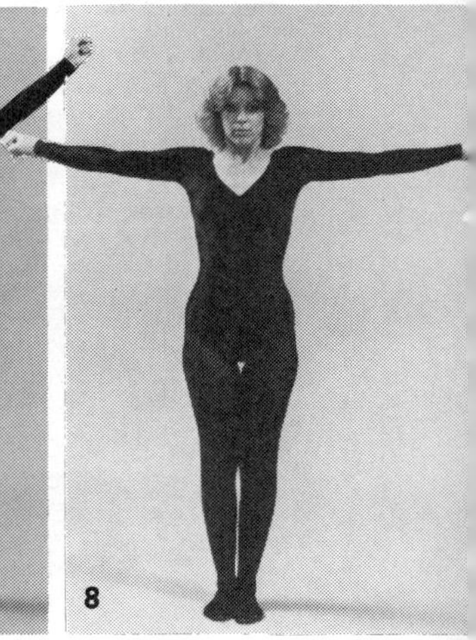

BACK EXERCISE #1

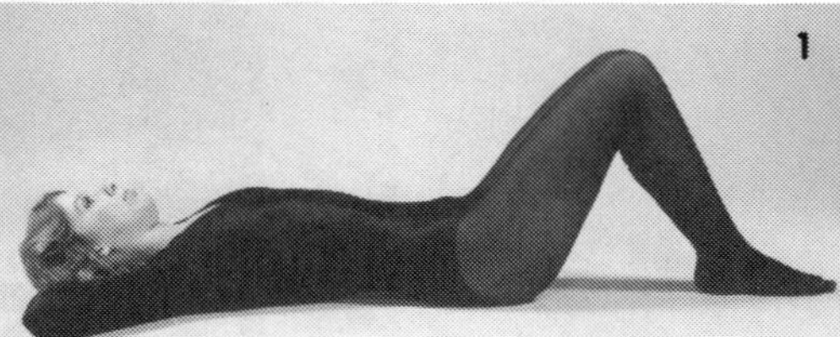

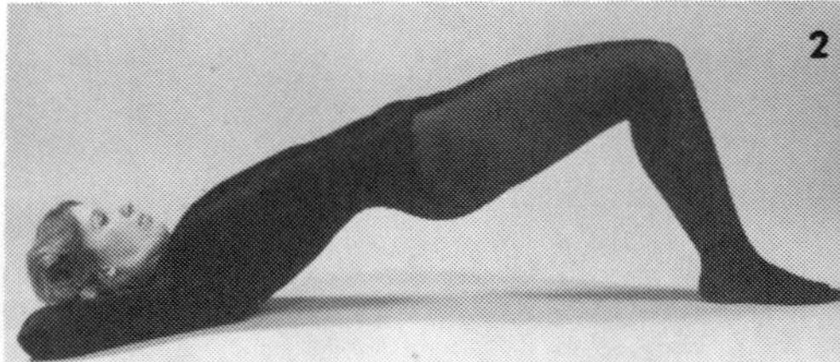

Lie on your back (1) with your knees bent and your hands clasped behind your head. Your feet should be flat on the floor. Then (2) flatten the small of your back and bring the lower end of your pelvis forward. Hold this position for a five-count and then (3) relax. Do this exercise ten times.

BACK EXERCISE #2

Begin (1) by lying on your back with your legs out straight. Then (2) grasp your raised right knee with both hands and (3) pull it as close to your chest as possible. Return it (4&5) to the starting position, and repeat the exercise with your other leg. Do this ten times for each leg.

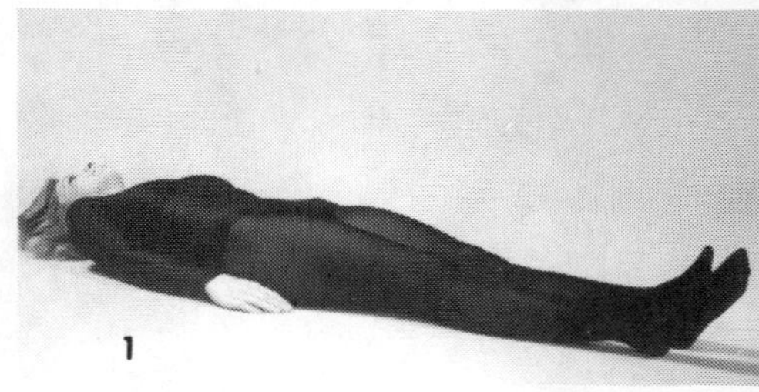

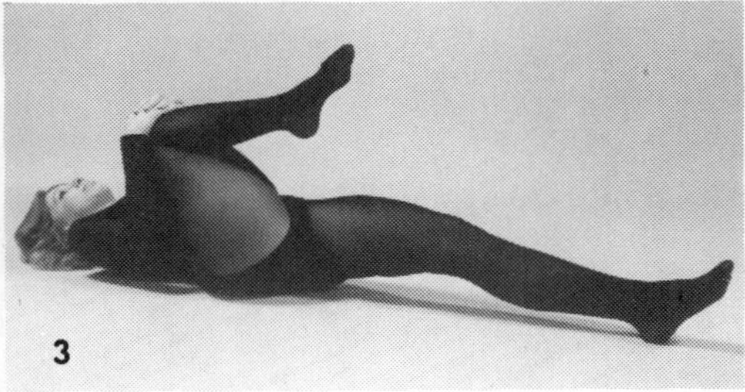

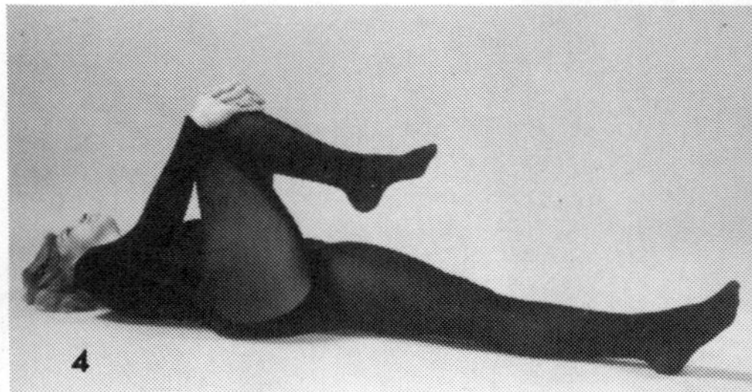

Lower back injuries can and do occur in martial arts activities and usually are mild strains and sprains in nature. Once pain and spasm in the injured area has lessened following ice application, gentle lower back exercises should be started on a daily basis. These exercises are designed to lessen spasm and increase flexibility of the lower back area. Mild aching may occur after performing the flexion exercises. If severe pain is present or begins during the exercises, they should be discontinued for up to four days, and ice should be applied.

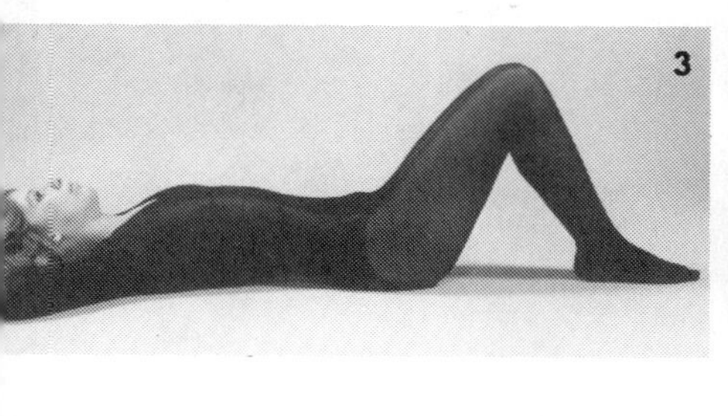

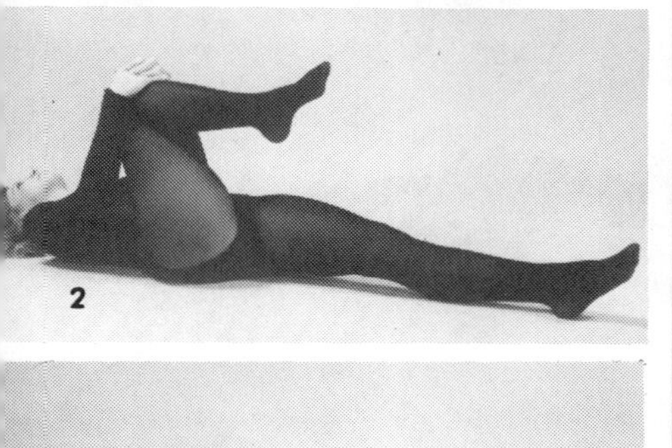

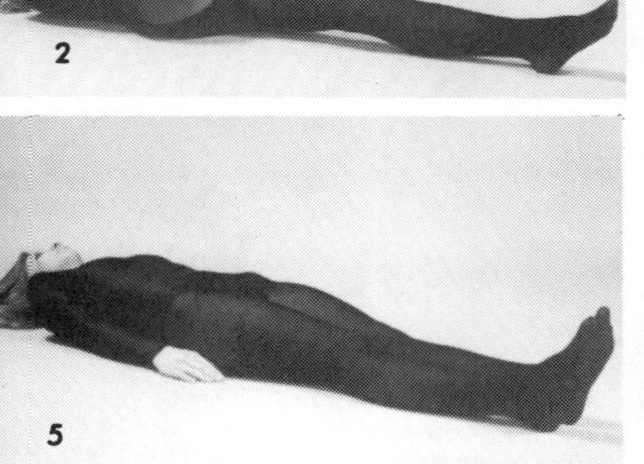

BACK EXERCISE #3

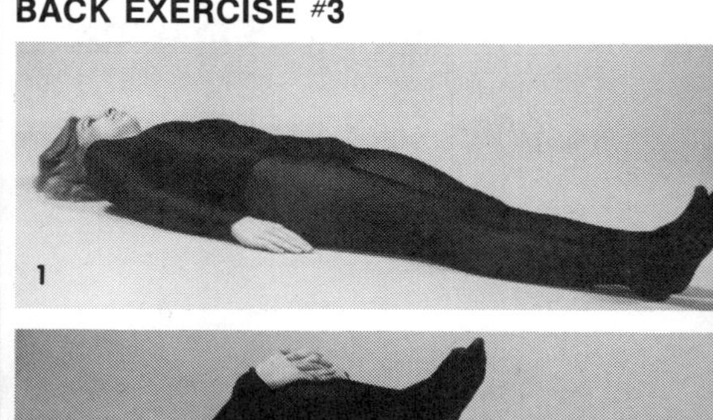

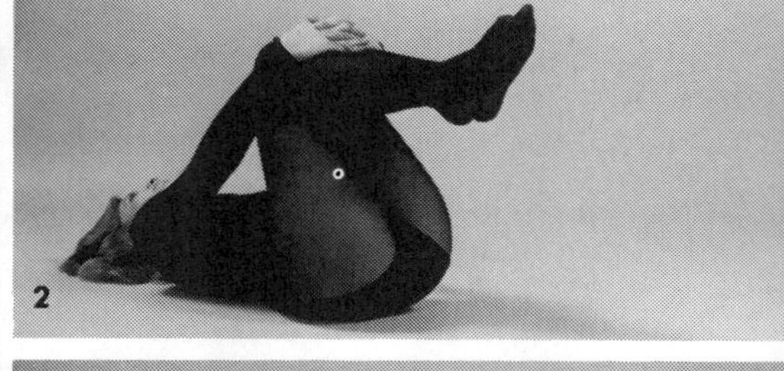

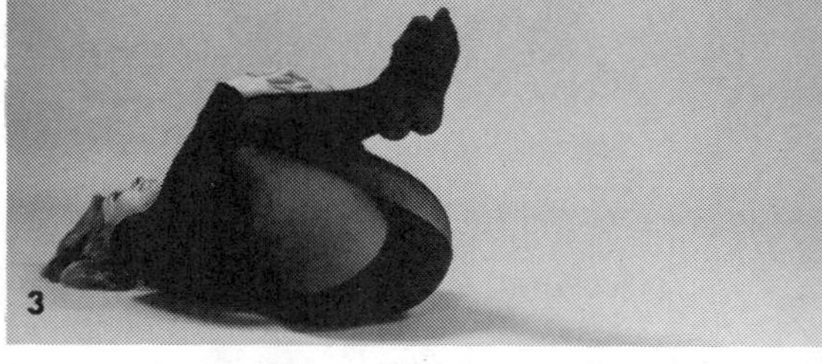

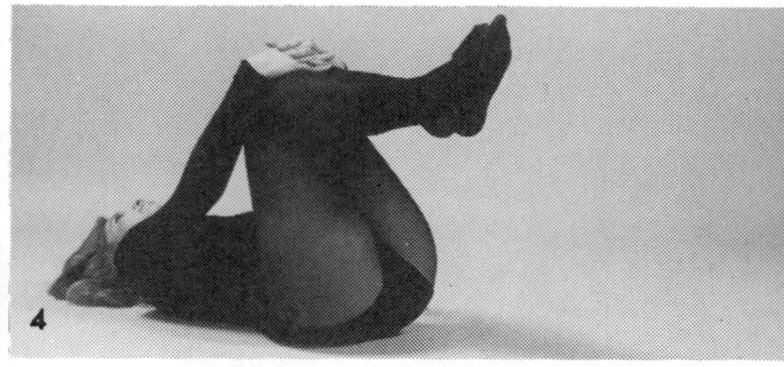

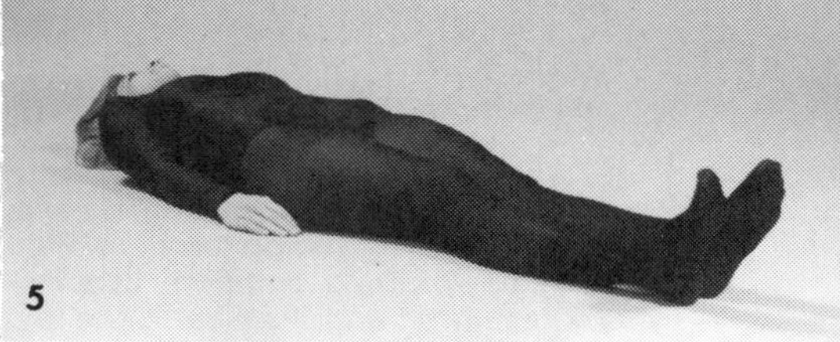

Assume the same starting position (1) as in exercise two. Then (2) grasp both knees and pull them (3) as close to your chest as possible. Hold the position, then (4&5) return to the starting position. Do this exercise ten times.

BACK EXERCISE #4

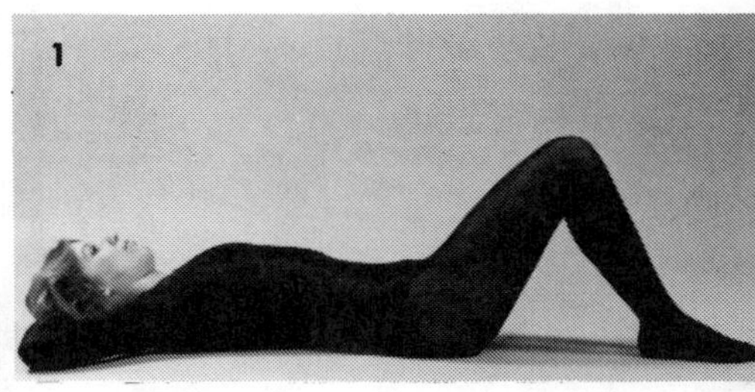

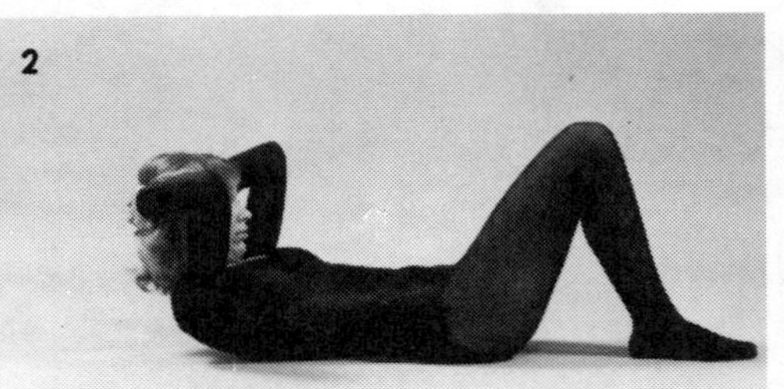

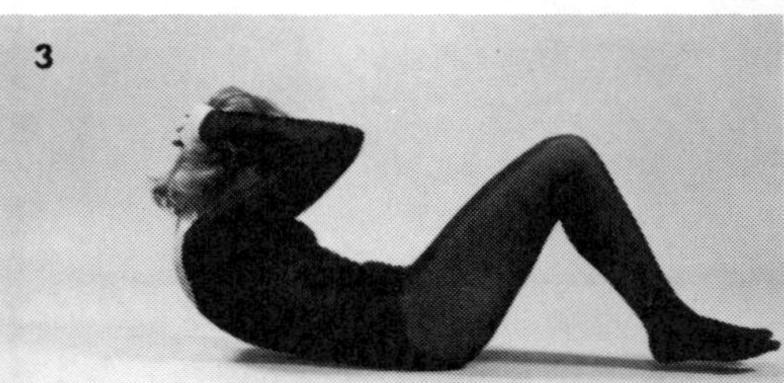

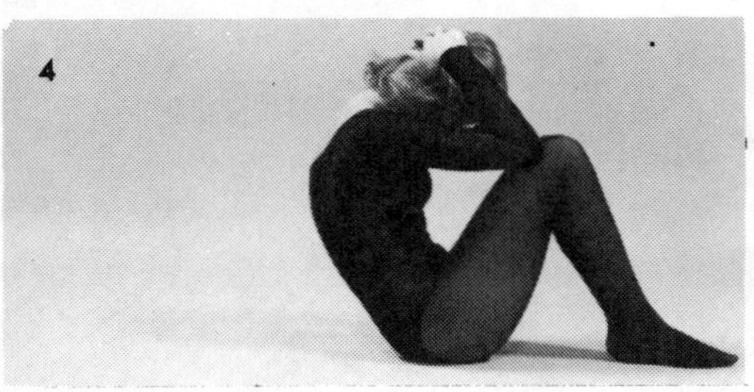

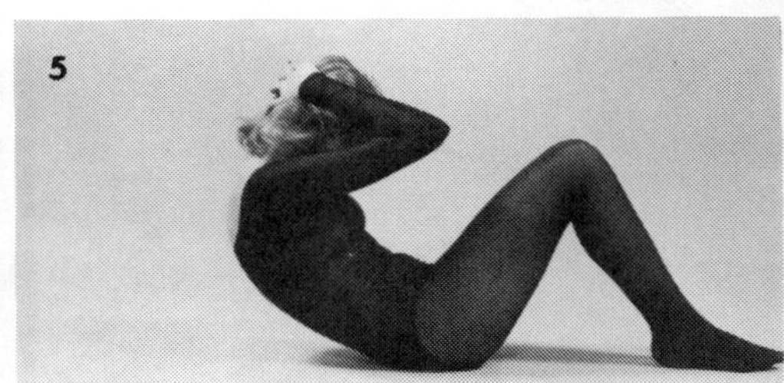

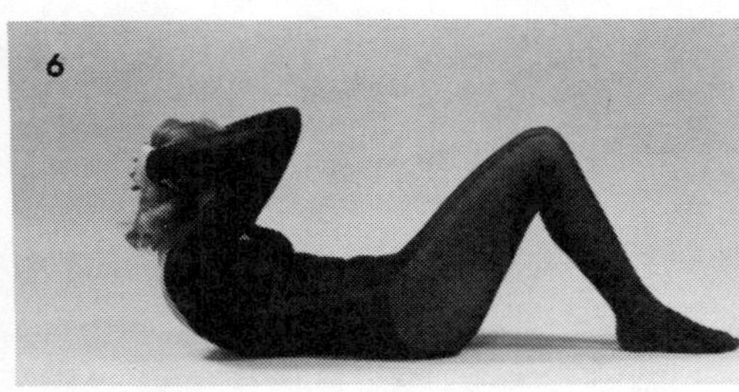

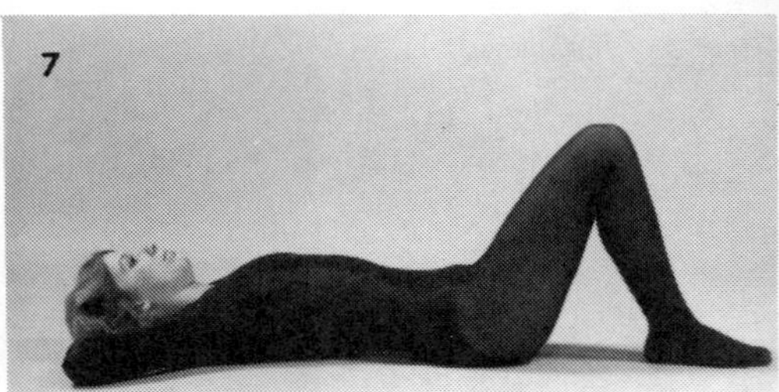

Lie on your back (1) with your knees apart and your feet flat on the floor. Pull up (2-4) to a sitting position, keeping your knees bent and your back slightly rounded. As you return to the lying position (5-7) keep your back flexed in a rounded position until your back touches the floor. (This avoids arching your back which can cause increased back strain.) Repeat the exercise ten to 15 times.

BACK EXERCISE #5

Lie on your back (1) with your legs out straight and your heels placed on an object 12-16″ off the floor. Then (2) thrust your pelvis upwards toward the ceiling so that your body is straightened and suspended between your heels and upper back. Hold this for one second then (3) relax and go back to the starting position. Do this 10-20 times per day.

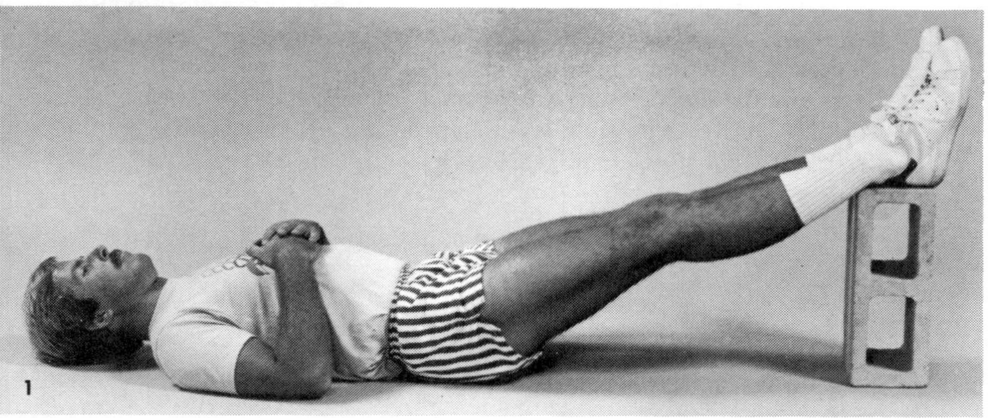

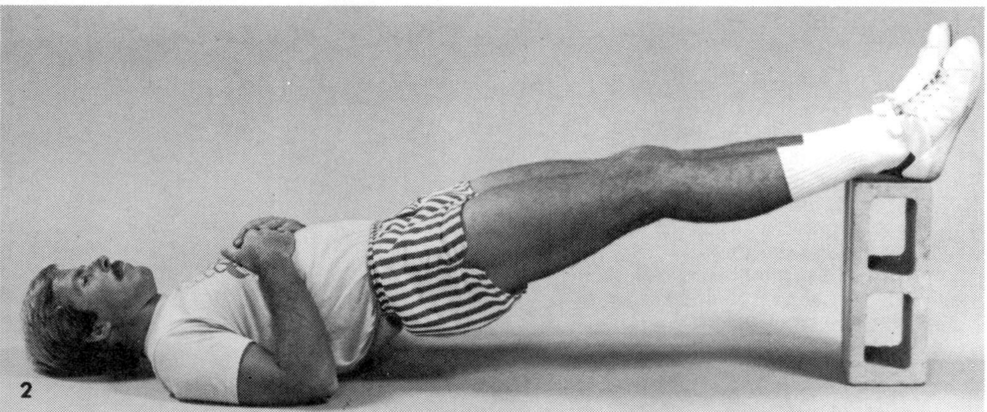

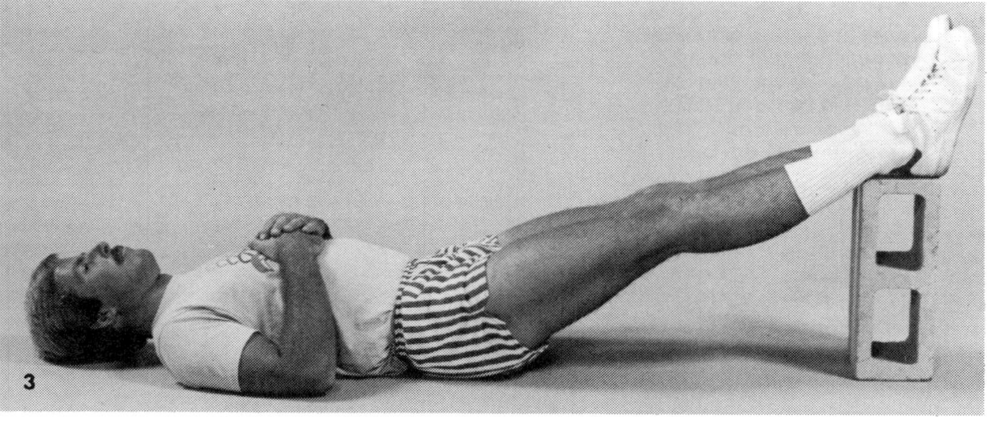

KNEE EXERCISES

When there is injury around the knee joint, there is neurogenic response which causes a decrease in muscle tone and strength of the muscles around the knee. Early institution of knee exercises decreases this response and restores normal muscle tone to the muscles affecting the knee. The quadriceps and the hamstring group supplies the major muscles of the knee. The rehabilitation exercises are designed to strengthen these muscles.

QUADRICEPS SITTING EXERCISE

Sitting on a flat surface, such as the floor, position your legs straight out in front of you. Tighten your knees by tensing the thigh muscles without moving the legs out of position. Hold the contraction for a ten-count and then relax. Continue this sitting exercise for three to five minutes. Best results are obtained if this can be done each hour during the day. This maneuver can also be done while sitting at work or in class or while driving.

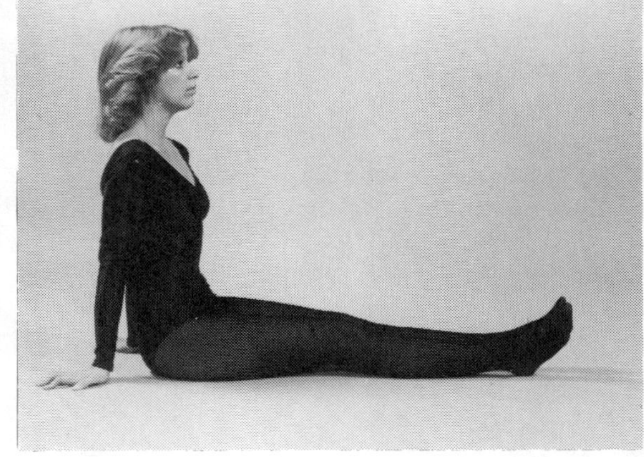

STRAIGHT LEG RAISES

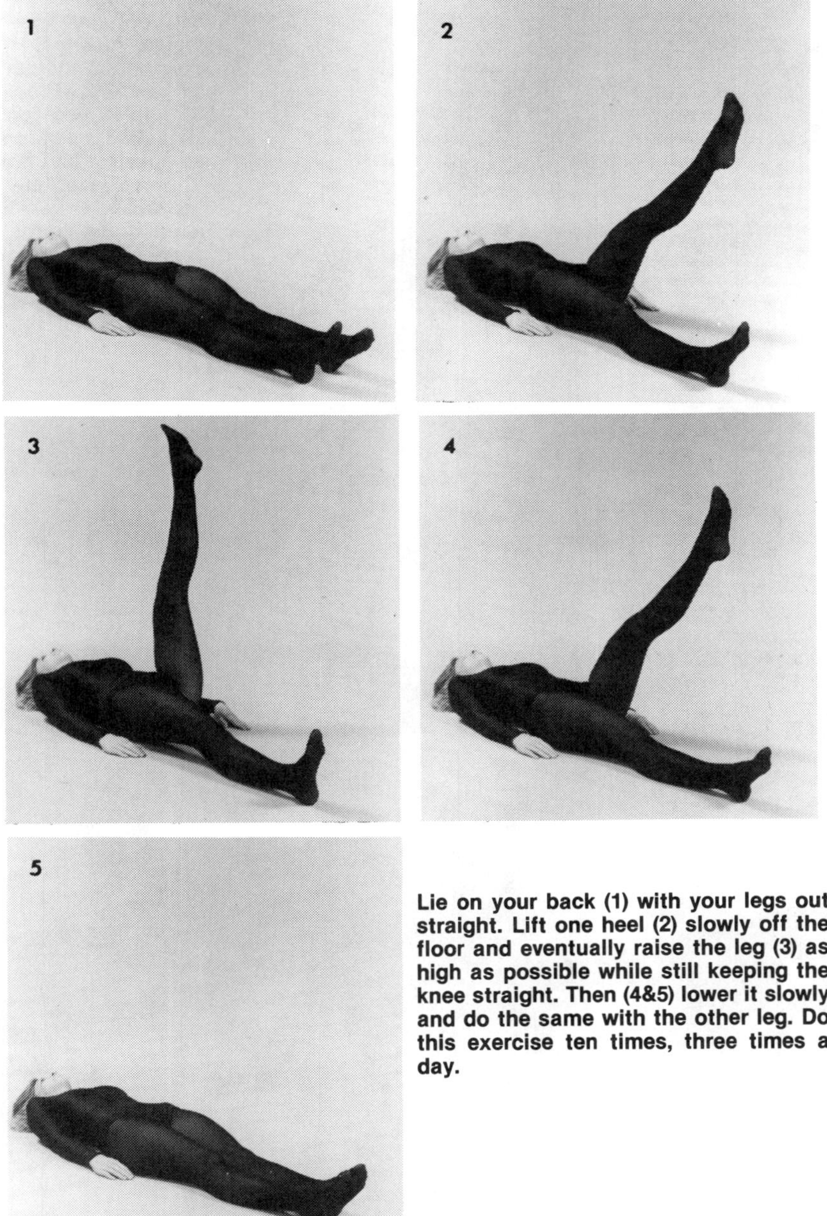

Lie on your back (1) with your legs out straight. Lift one heel (2) slowly off the floor and eventually raise the leg (3) as high as possible while still keeping the knee straight. Then (4&5) lower it slowly and do the same with the other leg. Do this exercise ten times, three times a day.

LEG EXTENSIONS

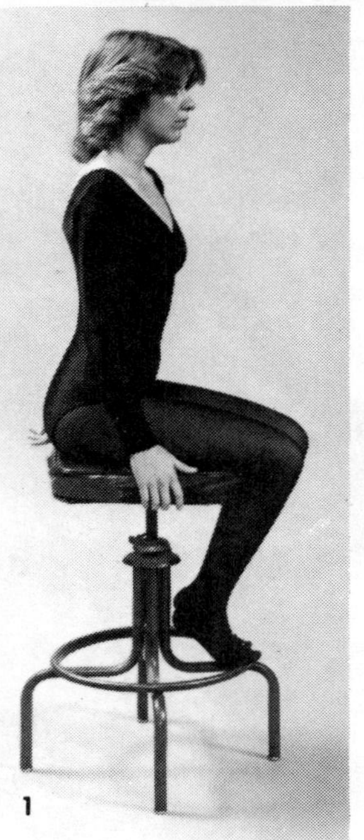

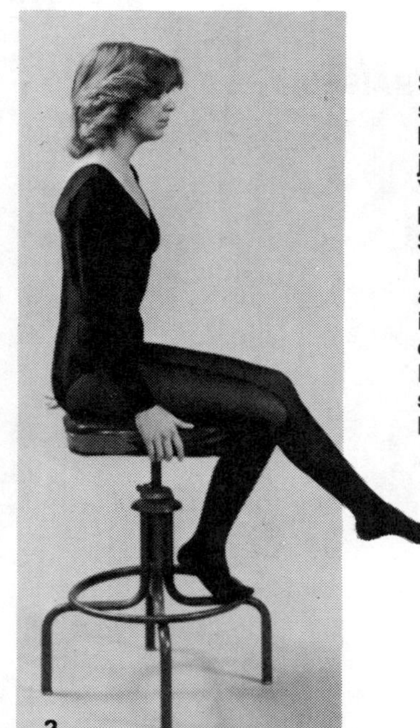

Sit on a high table or stool (1) with the backs of your knees just at the edge. Your knees should be bent and at rest. Straighten your left knee (2&3) as much as possible and hold it for a five- or ten-count, and then (4&5) lower it and do the same with the other leg.

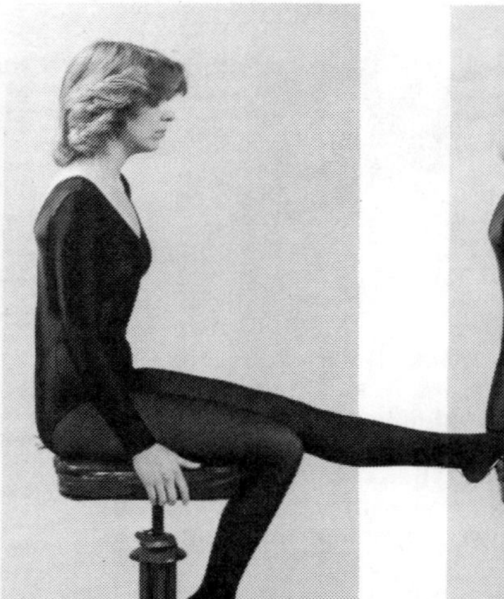

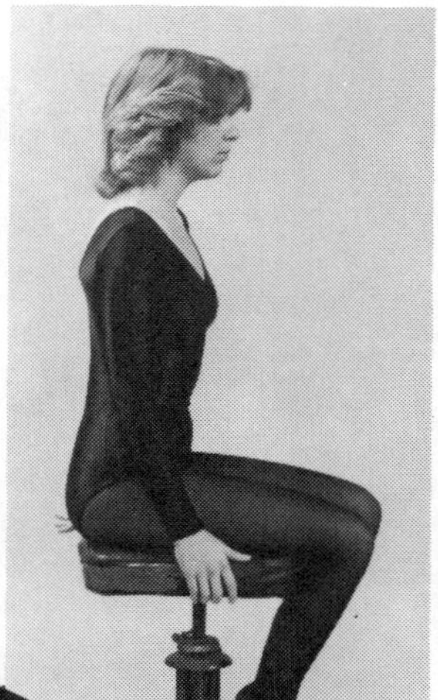

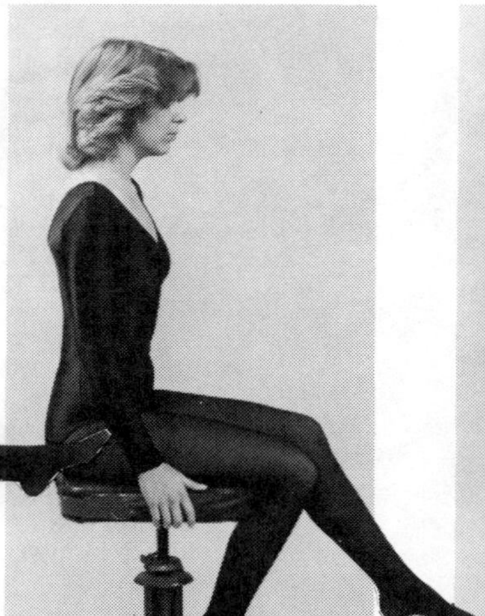

LEG EXTENSIONS WITH ANKLE WEIGHTS

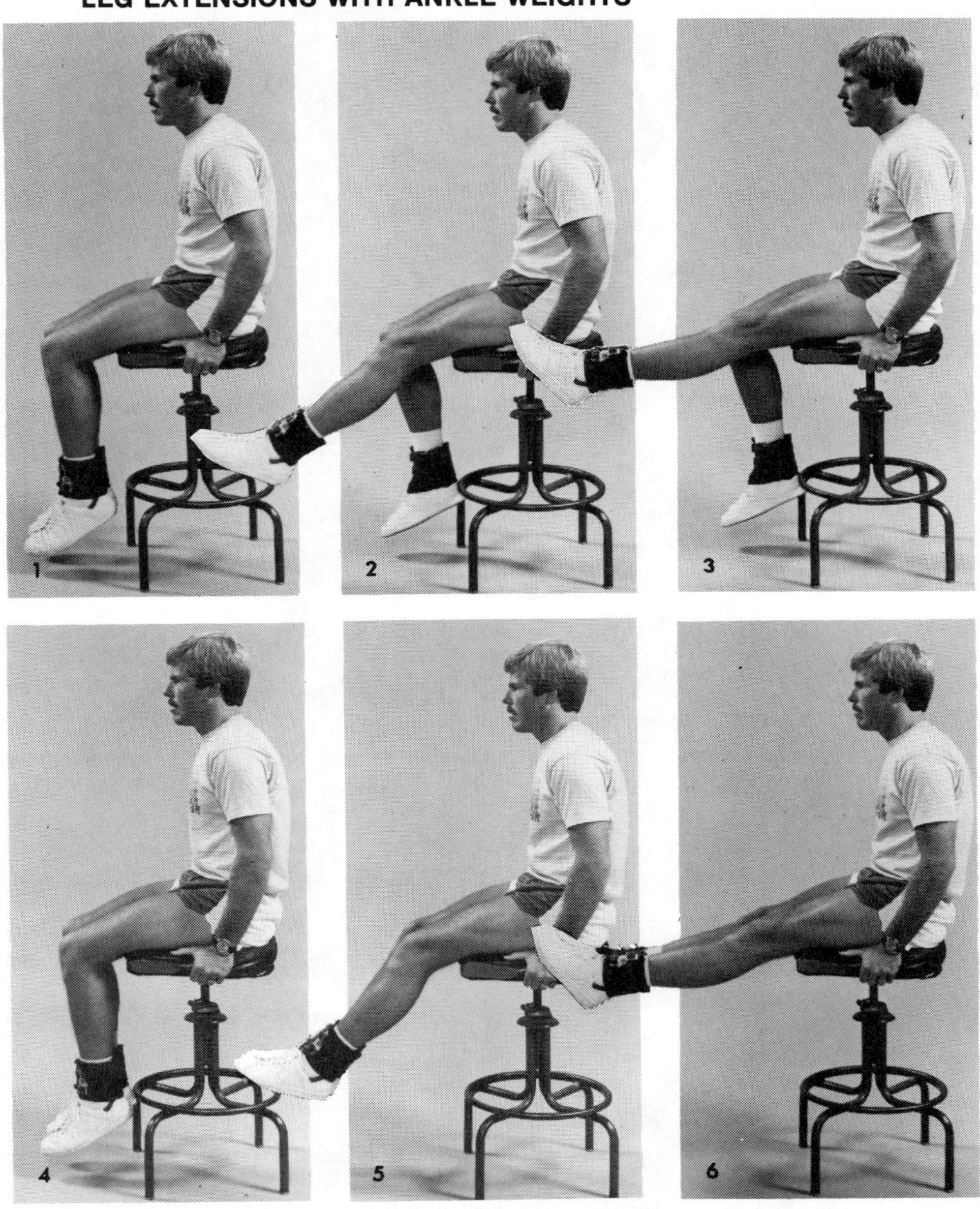

This exercise can be done with ankle weights (1-3) in order to build more strength in the knee. It should also be done (4-6) with both legs at the same time.

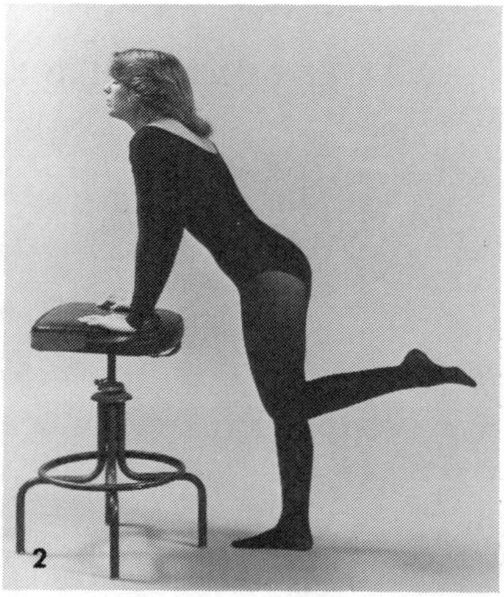

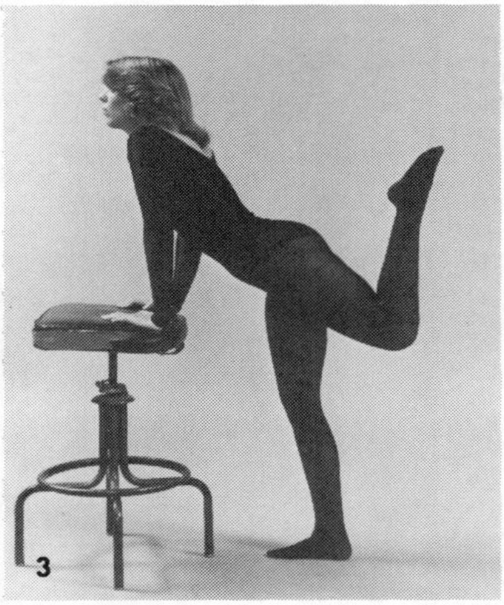

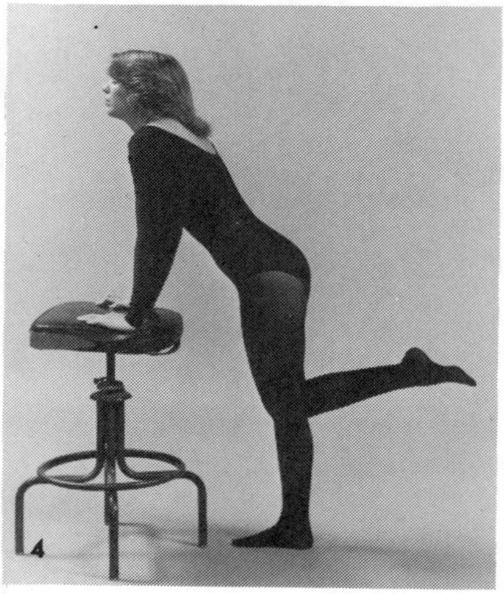

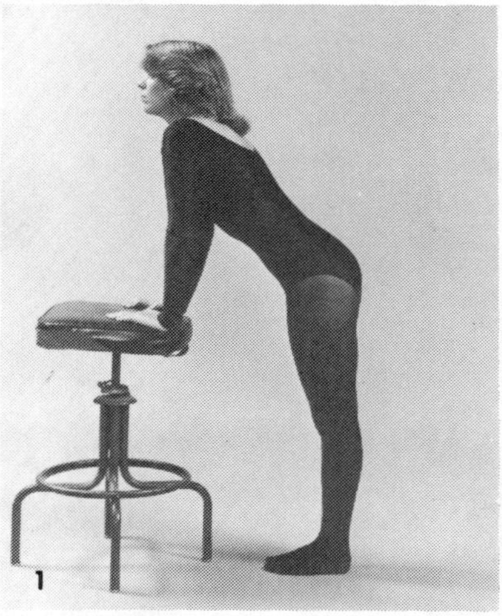

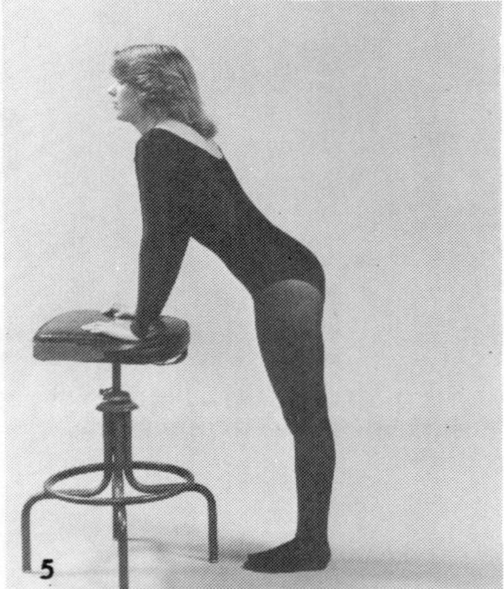

STANDING KNEE FLEXIONS

Stand (1) in front of a table or stool. Bend your left knee (2) and flex the leg (3) backward toward the back of the thigh. Relax (4&5) and lower the leg, then do it again with the other leg. Do this exercise 10-15 times. It strengthens the hamstring group of muscles which act as antagonists to the quadriceps.

These basic rehabilitation exercises for the neck, shoulder, back and knee are offered to aid in a more rapid recovery program. This is by no means a complete rehabilitation exercise program. These simple exercises can be done at home or in the gym and should aid the martial artist in returning sooner to regular work-out activities. ∎

CHAPTER 8
STRETCHING AND WEIGHT TRAINING

It is fairly well-established that there are five basic components for top physical performance:

1. Flexibility
2. Strength
3. Endurance
4. Speed
5. Coordination

All of these components are necessary for becoming an expert performer in the martial arts or in any athletic field.

The general conditioning programs used in martial arts training are based on hundreds of years of tradition and experience. They are, for the most part, successful in developing these five components for good physical performance.

It is not this book's intention to change these basic conditioning programs developed through the centuries by the masters. It is this book's intention, however, to point out that modern research and study in athletic conditioning has changed some of the traditional concepts. Let's look at some of these new ideas.

Flexibility is one of the most important attributes for martial arts. This is the ability to move the joint through its complete range of motion. Flexibility can only be improved and maintained by daily specific stretching exercises.

There are two basic types of stretching exercises. One is ballistic, or fast, stretching, and the second is static, or slow, controlled, stretching. Studies have revealed that static stretching offers several advantages over ballistic stretching: 1) There is less danger of over-stretching, which usually results in strains of the muscle tissue and tendons; 2) Less energy and work is required; 3) Static stretching eliminates soreness—in fact, it relieves soreness; and 4) It increases flexibility more than the ballistic method.

It is recommended that instructors use slow, static stretching only as the first portion of warm-ups before going to static stretching and stretch kicks. Major areas, such as the lower back, hips, hamstrings, trunk and the shoulders, should receive the most attention during this flexibility exercise time. The important point to be made here is that all stretching exercises at the beginning should be slow without bouncing or rapid rebound movements. These static flexibility exercises should be done in a series of ten movements with a count of 10 or 20 per movement for each major area.

Most instructors usually include stretching exercises such as forward bending, back bending, trunk twisting, front splits, hurdler's stretch,

REGULAR CURLS   FRONT VIEW

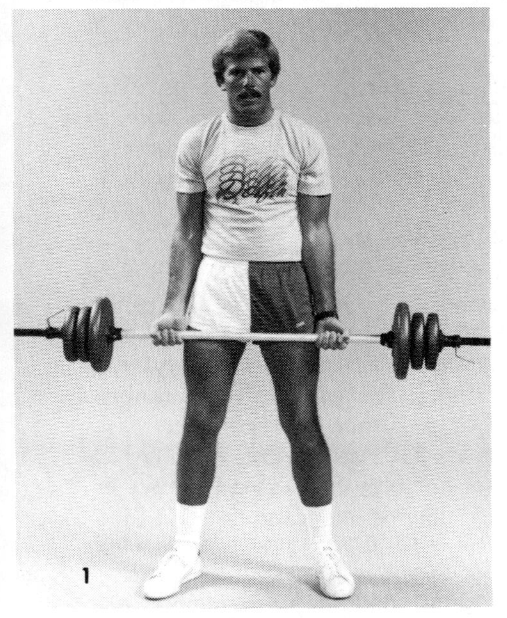

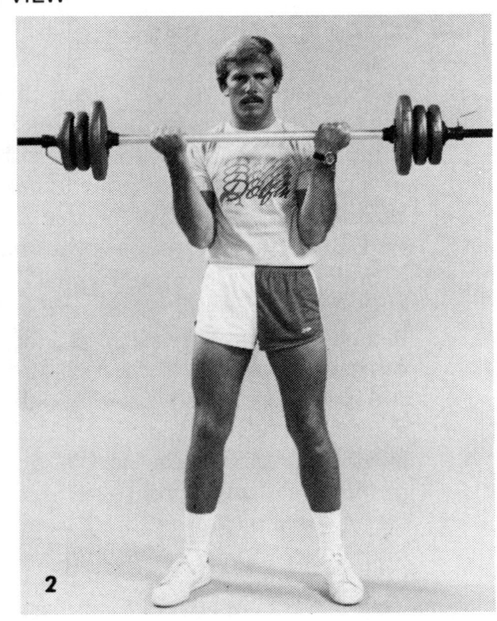

Do three sets of ten repetitions each day.

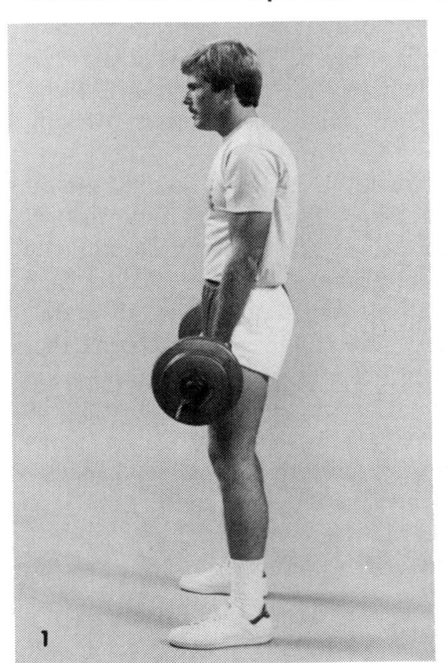

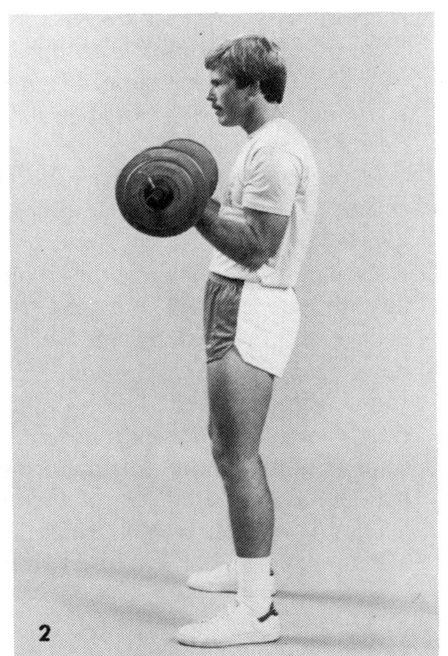

SIDE VIEW

shoulder circles, and so on. If these are done in the static manner, greater flexibility will be attained at a faster pace than fast, bouncing-type stretching.

After all the major areas and joints have been stretched, the instructor should move his students on to stretch-type kicks and floor exercises. It cannot be emphasized too much that strict attention must be paid to a proper warm-up period prior to moving on to the regular karate and judo exercises. This not only increases flexibility and cardio-pulmonary function, but it also reduces a great number of muscle and tendon injuries.

Strength development has had an almost revolutionary change since 1945. It was during this period that scientific studies and their application in a clinical setting revealed the value of weight training using progressive resistance exercises. Some well-known martial arts masters, surprisingly, still preach against the use of weight training. Their reason is that it causes a person to be slow and muscle bound. This, of course, is a complete falsehood. Studies over the past 30-plus years have proven conclusively that properly performed resistance exercises not only build strength, but increase speed of movement, increase flexibility of joints and improve functional use.

Recent studies by A. Jones have proved that proper use of weight-training results in a greater range of joint motion and flexibility. This has been shown to be a major factor in the reduction of athletic injuries. There is conclusive data that weight training actually increases speed of movement of the major muscle groups. This is, of course, desirable in all forms of martial arts. Because of this, it is highly recommended that progressive resistance exercises be used in martial arts training to improve strength, flexibility and speed.

Other forms of resistance programs are now available, and these are excellent for rapid strength development as well. Many dojo are now offering the Universal Gym set-up. This provides a multiple station-type assistance program where the amount of resistance can be selected for each large muscle group. These units have become very popular for high school, college and professional football teams. Another form of resistance that has been developed is the Nautilus. This unit is a very beneficial program for maximum strength development. It is designed for isolating the development of muscle groups in the most efficient manner in a very short span of training time. The major drawback for both the Universal and the Nautilus is the initial cost of the units and the space required.

Here is a basic weight training program for the martial arts student which will promote increased strength and power. This routine can be

HALF SQUATS

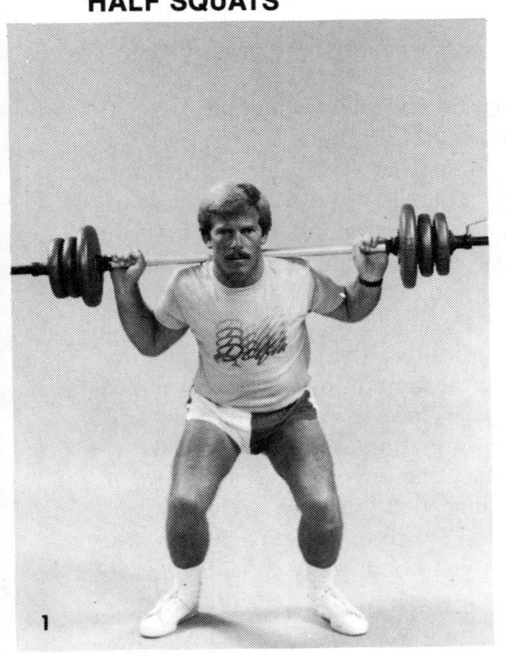

Do three sets of ten repetitions each day.

PRESS BEHIND THE NECK

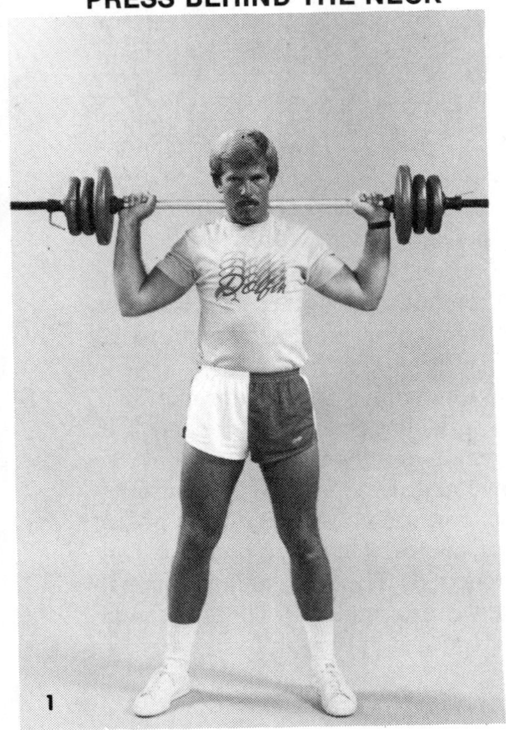

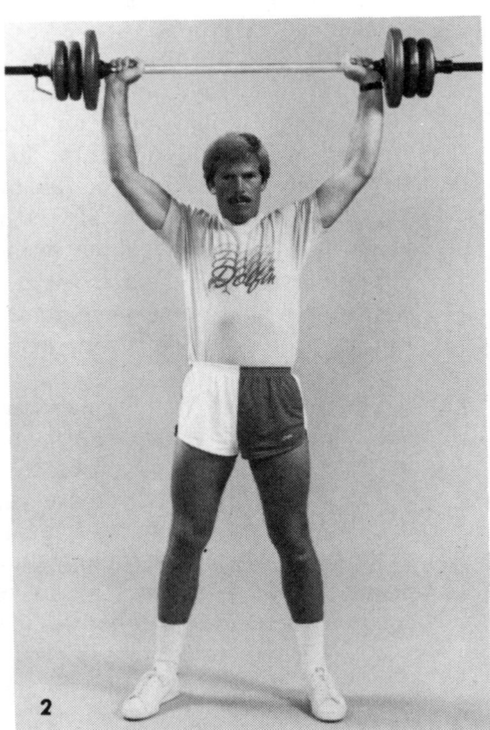

added to a regular karate training program and will produce great results in physical development as well as augment the martial arts skills. It is advised that weight training be done three days per week, such as Monday, Wednesday and Friday, or Tuesday, Thursday and Saturday. Heavy weights are not necessary when beginning weight training. Choose a weight that can be used for ten movements per exercise without excessive straining. Perform each exercise smoothly without jerking, allowing full extension of the joint and contracting to full flexion of the joint. Baer and his associates concluded after extensive studies that the major factor in improving muscular strength depended on the amount of tension developed by the muscle during exercises. Other studies have revealed that the faster a muscle contracts, the lesser the tension in it. Because of this, to develop strength in a muscle, a slower rate of contraction must be performed to develop the greater tension. It is recommended that each exercise movement not be too slow or too fast. If it takes two or three seconds to raise the weight, then it should take four or five seconds to lower it. Each exercise should be done through the full range of movement. If eight movements of an exercise cannot be performed in one set then the weight is too heavy. If one can perform 12 to 15 movements, the weight is too light. Larger muscle groups should be worked first, working down to the smaller muscle groups. At the beginning, only two sets of each exercise should be performed to avoid muscle soreness. Later, after 30 days of training, three sets should be done per each exercise.

The weight training program should ideally be done on the non-karate training days. If you train in the dojo on Tuesdays, Thursdays and Saturdays, then you should weight train on Mondays, Wednesdays and Fridays. This weight program could also be done after regular karate training, but it would be less beneficial due to the increased fatigue factor.

These seven basic exercises are given only as a basic routine to use when starting a weight-training program. There are many other exercises that can be incorporated into your weight-training program after eight to 12 weeks of basic work.

The basic weight training exercises in this manual are given primarily to develop general body strength for the beginning or average student. It is not intended as the total answer to strength development, however.

The martial arts masters have known and demonstrated for centuries that the waist and abdominal area is the basic source of strength and power of the body. Modern physiology studies have proven this to be a fact. Out of the studies have come three basic tenets: 1) The waist and abdominal region connects the upper body to the lower extremities; 2) The largest and

TOE RAISES

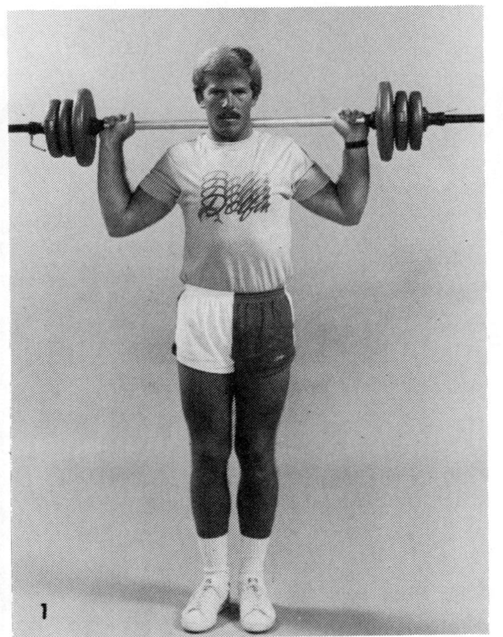 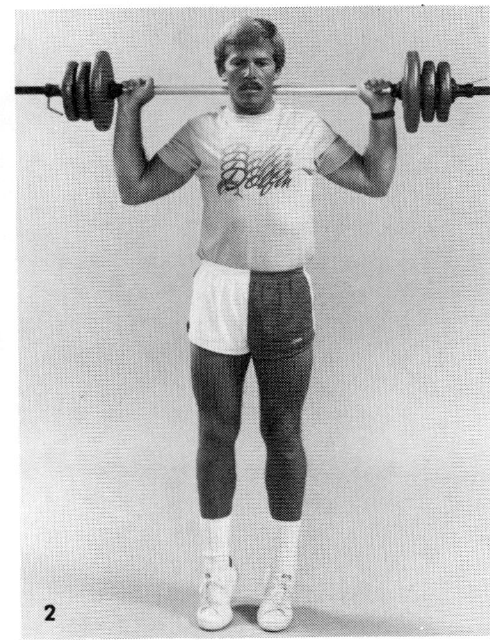

Do three sets of ten repetitions each day.

strongest muscles of the body are located in the abdominal lower back area and are connected to the pelvis; 3) The waist and abdominal area contain about one-third of the weight of the entire body.

Contrary to popular opinion, almost all athletic activities, especially in the martial arts, begin in the muscles at the body's center of gravity (the midsection). Therefore, resistance exercises that help develop the midsection and lower back are highly beneficial for the increased body power. Two exercises are recommended for this purpose. One is the bend-over twist using a rotational movement with one end of the barbell weighted with up to 50 pounds and the other end empty. The second exercise recommended is performing twisting set-ups with a barbell weighted on one end (beginning with about 15-20 pounds and working up to 75 pounds).

A.A. Steinhaus introduced the concept in 1963 that athletes can develop power in their particular sport by using a small resistance overload while

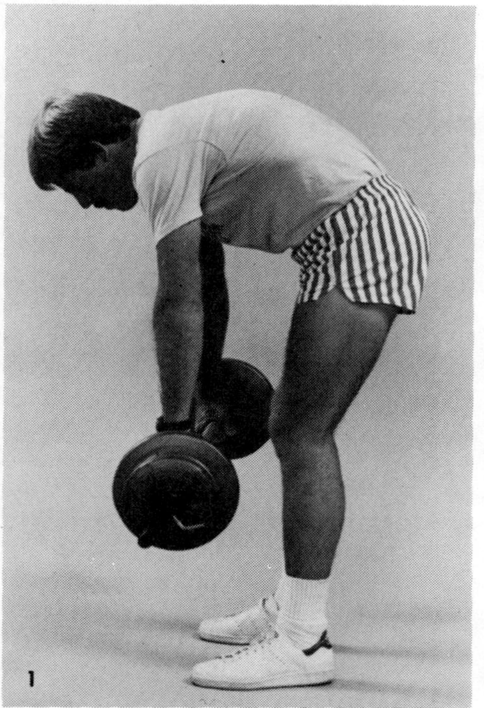
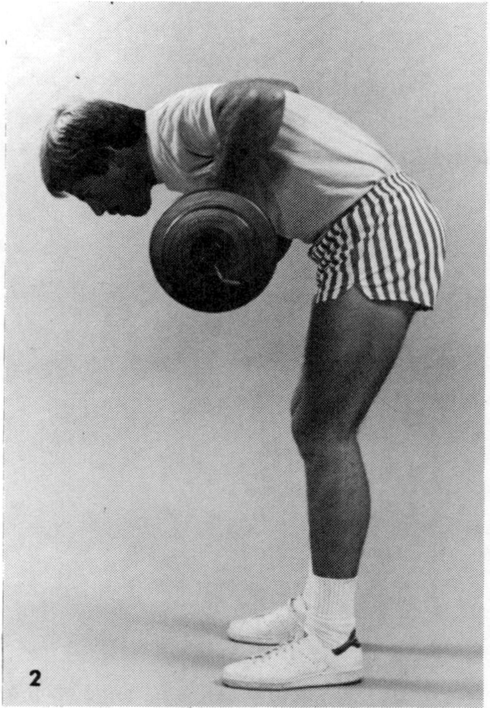

BENT-OVER ROWING MOTION

Do three sets of ten repetitions each day. You may want to support your head on a bench or table in order to avoid excessive strain on your lower back.

going through the motions used in that particular sport. In other words, he recommends using an overload shotput, discus or javelin for these specific sports. He recommended overweight bats for baseball players, leg weights for runners or jumpers, overweight basketballs or medicine balls for those ball players, and small 1-2½-pound barbells for boxers to hold in their hands while going through punching movements.

In the martial arts, the use of light one- to two-pound dumbbells or wrist weights for hand movements and five-pound dumbbells or wrist weights for hand movements and five-pounds ankle weights for kicking movements is highly recommended to develop increased power to karate. It is left up to the ingenuity and creativity of the individual instructor to develop his own exercises from the basic principles given in this manual.

THE BENCH PRESS

Use a wide grip and do three sets of ten repetitions every day.

1

2

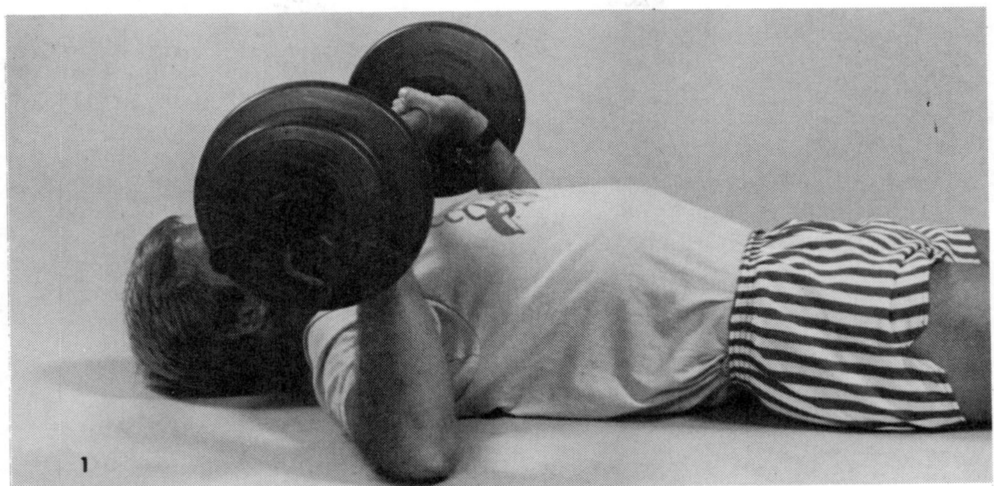

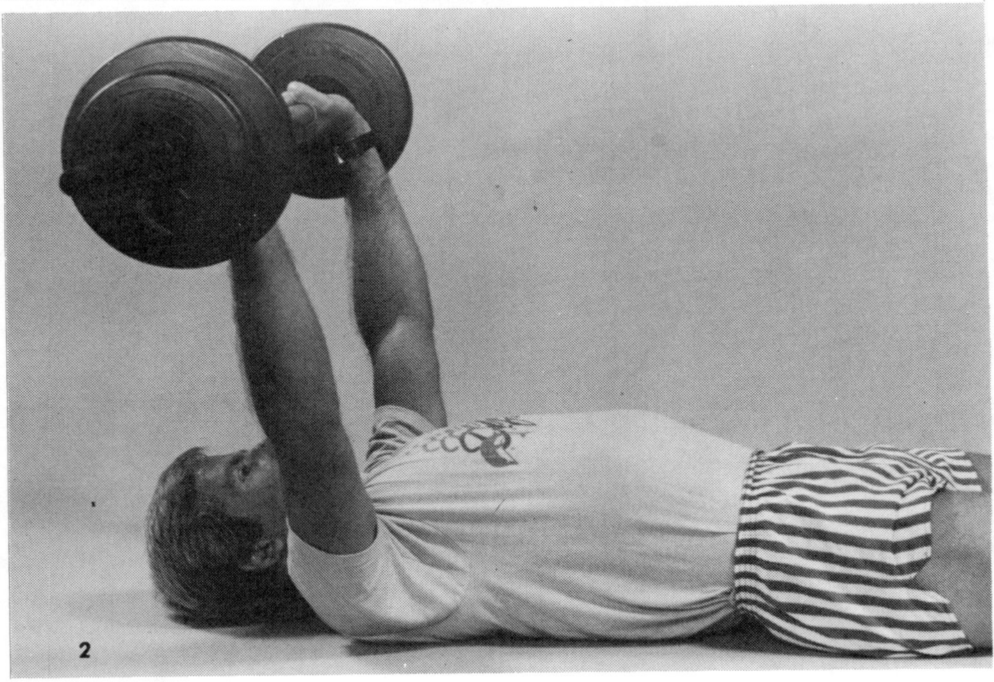